FRCS General Surgery Viva Topics and Revision Notes

STEPHEN BRENNAN

MBChB BSc (Pharm) MRCS (Ed) FRCSEd (Gen Surg)
Specialist Registrar in General Surgery
Raigmore Hospital, Inverness

Radcliffe Publishing
London • New York

Radcliffe Publishing Ltd
33–41 Dallington Street
London
EC1V 0BB
United Kingdom

www.radcliffepublishing.com

Electronic catalogue and worldwide online ordering facility.

British Library Cataloguing in Publication Data

A catalogue record for this book is available from the British Library.

ISBN-13: 978 184619 498 6

The paper used for the text pages of this book is FSC certified. FSC® (The Forest Stewardship Council®) is an international network to promote responsible management of the world's forests.

Typeset by Pindar NZ, Auckland, New Zealand
Printed and bound by TJ International, Padstow, Cornwall, UK

Contents

About the author

Stephen Brennan initially graduated in pharmacology and then studied medicine at the University of Aberdeen. He is currently a specialist registrar in general surgery with a particular interest in upper GI and laparoscopic surgery, and also trauma and the general surgery of childhood. In addition, he is involved with both undergraduate and postgraduate surgical training and is a tutor for the Royal College of Surgeons of Edinburgh and MRCS revision courses. He is an instructor in Advanced Trauma Life Support (ATLS) and has completed a postgraduate qualification in medical education.

Preface

FRCS General Surgery Viva Topics and Revision Notes is neither intended to be a textbook of surgery nor is it a guide for managing the surgical take. It is simply a collection of topics that tend to come up with regular frequency in the exam. As a surgical registrar who has recently passed the FRCS, my aim is to provide future candidates with a selection of ideas, exam tips, hints and suggestions, and advice that I received from my surgical trainers while preparing for this exam. The exit FRCS should be a once-in-a-lifetime experience and may well be the most stressful time in your life. These are my suggestions along the way.

My advice is to plan when you are going to sit the exam and just write the cheque. I sat the exam in year 5, but you should be at a stage where you could take out a colon, a gallbladder, or a spleen by yourself. Any sooner and you probably will not have seen or done enough to be confident to cover the scenarios they will give you in the viva with ease.

Part One is separated into chapters covering conditions that are common in the exam. I claim no expertise in any of them. This book is designed to be used in conjunction with some key textbooks that I feel are essential reading in order to pass this exam. First, I believe that the companion series should be the bible for the exam. You will need an up-to-date set and would be well advised to read them all cover to cover. The second book I believe is essential for the exam is *Emergency Abdominal Surgery*, edited by Jones, Krukowski and Youngson (3rd ed.; 1998). Unfortunately, it is out of print but contains the secrets of three surgical masters and will provide answers to situations that no other textbook will. Bailey and Love should be read cover to cover as all the examiners will have read it too.

Part Two of the book contains 120 multiple choice questions (MCQs), which are as close to the real thing as possible. They are based on actual questions from the exam that candidates recalled immediately thereafter. The remainder are designed de novo.

A further piece of advice is to do a preparatory or revision course. There are a few around and likely more to follow. It will cost you around £1500 for the week, so that with the exam fee itself, the books, travel and accommodation will leave you little change from £5K at the end of the day. That should be enough motivation to pass the first time!

A revision course is helpful, as it will not only test you on topics you possibly never thought about, it will also give you the necessary confidence to defend your answers under scrutiny. Remember this is a consultant's exam, and it is not sufficient to give a range of options. You must tell the examiner what you as a consultant are going to do.

The single most useful method of revision is simply going to work every day. Seeing patients in clinic and on-call is essential. This exam tests clinical management, not basic science. The EWTD and MMC do little to help the exam candidate here. Read your ATLS manual. Read the diathermy section of the basic surgical skills course.

Coming up to the exam, go to a variety of other specialty clinics. This means plastics, urology, orthopaedics, vascular and paediatric surgery. If you have declared general surgery for the exam, then you are fair game for melanomas, varicocoeles, hydatid of Morgagni, carpal tunnel syndrome, hernias and ingrown toenails. They are regularly examined. You must know the SIGN and NICE guidelines for everything.

The critical care viva needs an ITU anaesthetist to get you up to speed with inotropes and ventilators. Surgeons, if they are honest, know very little about these areas. You just need the basics for the exam. In the exam you need to be safe and will be expected to discuss the topics covered in this book.

The academic viva can be tackled by attending (or creating) a journal club each week for a couple of months prior to the exam. I would recommend reading the *British Journal of Surgery* for at least six months prior to the exam and ideally during the previous year. There is a high probability that at least one of the papers will be taken from there.

This book is divided into areas of general surgery that are common exam topics and not frequently studied. The suggested answers given here are by no means meant to be comprehensive but a guide to the key discussion points you should be prepared to discuss.

Stephen Brennan
April 2011

Acknowledgements

I wish to express my sincere gratitude to all my surgical trainers over the years. A few have stood out. Mr Norman Binnie for supporting me through thick and thin, Professor Ron Keenan for teaching me how to fix a hernia, Mr Keith Buchan for teaching me how to open a chest, Mr John Duncan for teaching me how to take out a gallbladder and, finally, to Mr Iain Gunn and Mr John Logie for inspiring me to become a surgeon in the first place.

For Kirsty

PART ONE

Vascular

> ➤ Abdominal aortic aneurysm (AAA)
> ➤ Varicose veins
> ➤ Acute and critical limb ischaemia
> ➤ Carotid disease
> ➤ Deep vein thrombosis

ABDOMINAL AORTIC ANEURYSM
What is an aneurysm?
An aneurysm is a permanent localised dilatation of an artery >50% diameter. The word comes from *aneurusma*, a Greek word meaning 'to widen'.

Most common sites of arterial aneurysm formation (in descending order)
- ➤ Infra-renal abdominal aorta.
- ➤ Popliteal.
- ➤ Femoral.
- ➤ Carotid.

Risks for aneurysm formation
- ➤ Male (6 times more common than females).
- ➤ Smoking (8 times more common).
- ➤ Genetic.
- ➤ Marfan's syndrome.
- ➤ Ehlers-Danlos syndrome Type 4.

NB: They are NOT related to 'berry' aneurysms.

Quoted figures
- ➤ 75% symptom-free when diagnosed (incidental).

➤ 75% mortality if AAA ruptures.
➤ 50% mortality if ruptured AAA reaches hospital.
➤ 25% AAA have synchronous lesion.

What is the evidence for elective repair at 5.5 cm?
UK Small Aneurysm Trial, *Lancet* 1998
➤ 1000 patients.
➤ 500 ultrasound surveillance (USS).
➤ 500 elective repair.
➤ 30-day mortality 5.8% (operative).
➤ No significant survival advantage at 6 years for AAA 4.0–5.5 cm.

What do you know about AAA screening?
The Highland Aneurysm Screening Project (HASP) based in Inverness demonstrated:
➤ screening the adult male population reduced the incidence of AAA rupture by 50%
➤ little benefit screening females.

AAA screening introduced in UK 2010
➤ Men aged 65 invited for one-off abdominal USS.

Supporting evidence: *BJS* (1994) showing that a single ultrasound scan at aged 65 will detect 90% AAA at risk of rupture.

What are the surveillance intervals?
UK AAA surveillance

5.5 cm	Elective repair
4.5–5.4 cm	Six-monthly scan
3.5–4.4 cm	Annual scan

What is EVAR?
Endovascular Aneurysm Repair
➤ Can be performed under GA or spinal anaesthesia.

Evidence
EVAR-1 trial, which was conducted in 1000 patients fit for open repair. The 30-day mortality was one-third less at 1.7% (versus 4.7%), with statistical significance $p = 0.009$.

Therefore all elective AAA repairs should be EVAR unless there are technical limitations preventing its use:

➤ neck <2 cm

➤ aneurysm/aorta angle >60 degrees.

What is an endoleak and how are they classified?

An endoleak is defined as persistent blood flow outside the graft within the aneurysm sac.

Type 1: Urgent repair as essentially ruptured aneurysm.

Type 2: Conservative management as low-pressure leak.

Type 3: Requires repair.

Type 4: Conservative management as leak contained (rare and therefore debatable).

What pre-op investigations would you perform for an elective AAA repair?

➤ FBC, UE, LFTs, coagulation screen, glucose, HbA1c if diabetic, lipids.

➤ Crossmatch 4 units.

➤ ECG.

➤ CXR.

➤ CT angiogram abdominal aorta.

➤ Exercise tolerance test/thallium.

➤ MUGA or ECHO (varies between units).

➤ ABG.

How would you repair a ruptured AAA?

The key manoeuvre in a ruptured AAA is converting an unstable case into an elective repair.

Key treatment steps

➤ Decision to operate in the first place.

➤ Consent with patient and relatives.

➤ Mobilise experienced theatre team.

➤ Initiate major transfusion protocol and ensure blood products available.

➤ Anaesthetic set-up: central line right internal jugular, arterial line, and urethral catheter. Anaesthetic agents to be administered only when surgeon ready.

➤ Prep and drape.

➤ Rapid opening of abdomen via long midline incision.

➤ Eviscerate small bowel and dissect duodenum to right.

➤ Proximal control of AAA neck:

   ➣ infra-renal: divide left renal vein

   ➣ supra-renal: split right crus of diaphragm/split lesser omentum for supra-coeliac control.

➤ Cross clamp on.

➤ Iliac control, then proceed as for elective repair.

What are the complications of AAA repair?

Complications may be classified as general and specific.

General
➤ Embolus.
➤ Thrombus.
➤ Cardiac.
➤ Respiratory/ARDS.
➤ Acute tubular necrosis.
➤ Ischaemic gut (IMA).

Specific
➤ Graft sepsis.
➤ Renal infarction.
➤ Gut ischaemia (IMA).
➤ Wound infection.
➤ Stroke.
➤ Incisional hernia.

How would you manage a post-op AAA who developed metabolic acidosis?

Causes
1 Acute tubular necrosis.
2 Ischemic left colon.
3 Abdominal compartment syndrome.

How would you do a brachial embolectomy?

➤ Heparin 5000 units IV.
➤ GA/local with anaesthetist present.
➤ Transverse incision at antecubital fossa.
➤ Split bicipital aponeurosis. **NB: Median nerve is medial to artery.**
➤ Proximal and distal control of brachial artery.
➤ Transverse arteriotomy (11 blade and Potts scissors).
➤ Embolectomy with size 3 and 4 Fogarty catheter.
➤ Heparin flush.
➤ 6/0 Prolene closure.
➤ Start warfarin post-op.

How would you manage a popliteal artery aneurysm?

Surgical therapy

Popliteal artery occlusion

Surgical therapy for popliteal artery occlusion is bypass of the occlusion, which can be achieved with grafts, including great saphenous vein (GSV) or prosthetic (e.g. polytetrafluoroethylene [PTFE]) grafts. GSV bypass can be used in a reversed, nonreversed or in situ orientation. The reverse vein bypass graft, first described by Kunlin in 1949, has become the favoured operation for bypass of an occluded popliteal artery. The ipsilateral GSV is the conduit of first choice. If that is unavailable, alternative autogenous conduit options that can be used include the contralateral GSV, arm veins (basilic and cephalic), the small saphenous vein, the superficial femoral vein, the popliteal vein, or cryopreserved veins.

The popliteal artery is accessible from medial thigh and calf incisions. The anastomosis can be performed either end-to-end or side-to-side. If the latter is chosen in the case of an aneurysm, the aneurysm must be excluded from the circulation by ligature.

Percutaneous transluminal angioplasty (PTA) is a less invasive intervention in the treatment of popliteal artery occlusive disease. PTA is indicated for short (<2 cm) lesions in patients who have claudication and good runoff. Initial enthusiasm that stents could increase long-term results of PTA has not been supported by subsequent studies. The primary patency rate at 1 year is 65%. However, PTA may be a reasonable alternative to open surgery for limb salvage indications in patients with prohibitive surgical risks.

Popliteal artery aneurysm

Elective surgical repair is indicated in all patients with PAA regardless of size. Even a small PAA can produce limb-threatening ischemia secondary to thrombus or distal embolisation. Elective repair assures that procedure is not performed in the setting of limb-threatening ischemia. Elective repair is associated with little risk to the patient, better overall results and lower incidence of amputation. Surgical PAA repair consists of either resecting the aneurysm sac or interposing a bypass graft or proximal and distal ligation of the popliteal artery combined with bypass grafting.

More recently, endovascular repair with a percutaneously delivered covered stents (stent grafts) has become an alternative to open repair, but long-term results are unknown.

Emboli

Emboli may be evacuated from distal vessels by either the use of a balloon catheter or intraoperative thrombolysis.

Popliteal entrapment syndrome

Surgical treatment is advised in all types of popliteal entrapment syndrome. Recognition of progressive fibrosis with subsequent thrombosis in untreated entrapped artery supports early surgical intervention. Individual anatomic considerations play an important role in determining the best surgical approach. Although the posterior approach has been most commonly advised because it most clearly delineates the anatomy of the lesion, the medial calf approach is more appropriate when the occlusion extends distally to the popliteal artery bifurcation. Myotomy of the compressing muscle or transection of fascial band leads to decompression of the artery and prevention of secondary fibrotic changes. If the artery is not occluded and fibrotic change has not occurred, no further intervention is necessary.

Recent evidence emerged that suggests when a popliteal artery has undergone fibrotic changes and occlusion, resection and vein graft (preferably GSV) interposition are required to ensure optimal long-term patency in these often young, physically active individuals.

Preoperative details

Most patients with occlusion of the popliteal artery have some component of CAD or another comorbid condition. Therefore, patients' current functional status must be taken into consideration. Preoperative ECG, chest radiography and coagulation studies are recommended. In non-emergent cases, performing lower extremity angiography is important for identifying the site of occlusion, any collateral circulation, and possible target vessels for bypass and for visualisation of runoff vessels. If the use of a vein is anticipated, duplex studies should be performed to assess the calibre and patency of the veins.

Those patients with gangrene of the affected leg require a course of antibiotics and wound care prior to the bypass operation. Although not an absolute contraindication, leg infections increase the incidence of graft infections and subsequent failure.

Intraoperative details

Careful cardiac monitoring must be used in the operative intervention of popliteal artery thrombosis. These patients usually have significant comorbid conditions (e.g. CAD, chronic obstructive pulmonary disease) that increase the risk of stroke, myocardial infarction, or bleeding episodes. Upon completion of the bypass, some form of confirmation of technical competency must be performed (e.g. completion angiography, intraoperative duplex US, continuous-wave Doppler US).

Postoperative details

On the first postoperative day, patients should begin aspirin therapy and, if indicated, beta-blockers. Postoperative ABI should be obtained before the patient is discharged from the hospital. These serve as a baseline to which subsequent ABISs can be compared in the event of restenosis. Postoperative visits for duplex scanning of the graft are undertaken every 3 months for a year and every 6 months thereafter.

Follow-up

Follow-up should be performed at regular intervals to assess for restenosis, which usually results from technical failures, intimal hyperplasia, or disease progression at other sites, at 1 month, 18 months, and 2 years or more, respectively.

VARICOSE VEINS

What is the epidemiology of varicose veins?
➤ Varicose veins are abnormal tortuous dilated superficial veins of the legs.
➤ 95% are primary (cf. DVT, occlusion).
➤ Affects approx. 20% population.
➤ Female > male (5:1) present.

Edinburgh vein study (1999): 40% male, 30% female, 18–64 years
➤ Which system is affected?
   ➢ Long or short?
➤ What is the state of SFJ?
   ➢ Competent or incompetent?
➤ What is the state of other perforators?
   ➢ AK, BK, ankle?
➤ What is the state of the deep system?
   ➢ Patent and competent or not?
➤ Complications?
   ➢ Pigmentations, ulcers?

Vascular clinic assessment
➤ History and examination.
➤ Brodie-Trendelenberg test.
➤ HHD.
➤ Duplex scan.
➤ Grade 2 below-knee compression hosiery.

What are the complications?
➤ Haemorrhage.
➤ Thrombophlebitis.
➤ Oedema.
➤ Skin pigmentation.
➤ Varicose eczema.
➤ Lipodermatosclerosis.
➤ Venous ulceration.
➤ DVT is NOT a complication.

What are the treatment options?
➤ Reassurance.
➤ Stockings (20–30 mmHg at ankle).
➤ HSL, strip and avulsions (day-case).
➤ Foam sclerotherapy.
➤ Laser therapy (EVLT).
➤ CLASS trial in progress.

Surgical complications
- Recurrence (20–35%)
- Nerve damage (4–25%)
- Haematoma (30%)
- Wound infection (2–15%)
- DVT (<2%)
- PE (0.2%).

Endovenous laser treatment (EVLT) versus foam sclerotherapy?
EVLT
- Performed in DCU.
- LA.
- Ultrasound-guided Seldinger technique.
- Shorter recovery time.
- Less discomfort.
- Less scarring.
- EVLT causes thermal damage of the vein wall, resulting in destruction of the intima, subsequent collagen denaturation of the media and fibrotic occlusion of the vein wall.
- Short-term efficacy and safety are similar compared to surgery.

Foam sclerotherapy
- Outpatient procedure.
- Butterfly needle 1% Fibro-vein (STD).
- Technical success rate 85%.
- Phlebitis/discoloration.
- Allergy/anaphylaxis.
- DVT 1%.
- Stroke (single case)/retinal artery occlusion.

ACUTE AND CRITICAL LIMB ISCHAEMIA
Define critical limb ischaemia
A critically ischaemic leg is defined as rest pain present for >2 weeks and/or tissue loss/necrosis.

How would you do a femoral embolectomy?
- Heparin 5000 units IV.
- GA.
- Vertical groin incision at mid-inguinal point.
- Lateral to medial dissection to avoid lymphatics.
- Proximal and distal control of femoral artery.
- Transverse arteriotomy (11 blade and Potts scissors).
- Embolectomy with size 3 and 4 Fogarty catheter.
- Heparin flush.

➤ 6/0 Prolene closure.
➤ Start warfarin post-op.

How would you manage a 25-year-old male with axillary vein thrombosis?

This condition is relatively rare. It usually presents in young and otherwise healthy patients, males more often than females. The syndrome also became known as 'effort-induced thrombosis' in the 1960s, as it has been reported to occur after vigorous activity, though it can also occur spontaneously. Symptoms include sudden onset of pain, warmth, redness, blueness and swelling in the arm. These DVTs should be treated as an emergency, but rarely cause fatal PE.

Treatment

The traditional treatment for thrombosis is the same as for a lower extremity DVT, and involves anticoagulation with heparin (generally low molecular weight heparin) with a transition to warfarin.

Management of a groin abscess in an IVDA

Severe vascular complications are rare but if they occur, therapy is difficult and requires emergency management and surgery because of bleeding problems.

Abscess excision and debridement have to be as complete as possible and primary revascularisation is the procedure of choice in cases of severe groin infection. In the case of large vessel involvement, abscess incision alone without revision of the vascular structures is dangerous because of subsequent complications like secondary ruptures. For this reason, these patients require intensive care and close monitoring. Successful treatment exclusively based on ligation is described in literature with regard to isolated lesions of the superficial or deep femoral artery. Because of the very common involvement of the femoral bifurcation, revascularisation is, however, necessary in most cases and should be performed with autologous grafts if possible. If complete covering of the defect is not possible, a sartorius muscle flap is a good choice. Primary wound closure can be problematic because of recurrences; therefore, vacuum-assisted wound closure is a valuable addition to the overall therapeutic approach in these cases.

CAROTID DISEASE

Carotid surgery

➤ European Carotid Surgery Trial (ECST): >80% stenosis, NNT = 12.
➤ North American Symptomatic Carotid Endarterectomy Trial (NASCET): >70% stenosis, NNT = 5.
➤ Vascular surgery society guidelines recommend carotid scan and surgery within 2 weeks.

➤ Asymptomatic Carotid Surgery Trial (ACST) showed benefit for male patients with NNT = 17.

DEEP VENOUS THROMBOSIS
What are the latest NICE guidelines on DVT prophylaxis?

NICE guideline CG92 (January 2010) has suggested that all patients admitted to hospital should be screened for DVT risk. Patients are scored for risks of both bleeding and DVT and their prophylaxis is determined according to this.

Factors for risk of bleeding

➤ Active bleeding present.
➤ Liver failure.
➤ On anticoagulants with INR >2.
➤ Lumbar puncture.
➤ Thrombocytopenia <75.
➤ Uncontrolled hypertension.
➤ Haemophilia.
➤ Von Willebrand's disease.

If any of the above conditions are present then the patient should get TEDS stockings only and not heparin.

If the patient has any of the following and no risks for bleeding, then he/ she should be managed with mechanical DVT prophylaxis, such as TEDS or flowtron boots +/– low molecular weight heparin (LMWH) and ideally for up to 5–7 days post discharge:

➤ total surgery time >90mins or
➤ pelvic/limb surgery >60mins or
➤ acute surgical admission or
➤ any of the following DVT risk factors:
    ➤ malignancy
    ➤ age >60 years
    ➤ HDU admission
    ➤ dehydration
    ➤ thrombophillia
    ➤ BMI >30
    ➤ oral contraceptive pill
    ➤ HRT
    ➤ varicose veins with phlebitis
    ➤ comorbidity such as cardiac failure.

Hepatobiliary

> Jaundice
> Liver function tests (LFTs)
> Mirizzi's syndrome
> Hepatocellular carcinoma (HCC)
> Pancreatic carcinoma
> Sphincter of Oddi (SOD) dysfunction
> Gallbladder cancer and gallbladder polyps
> Acute cholecystitis
> The spleen
> Acute pancreatitis
> Benign liver lesions

JAUNDICE
Explain bile production and metabolism
Bile consists of:
> products for excretion:
>> bile pigments (red blood cells)
>> cholesterol (fat metabolism)
>> fat-soluble drugs and toxins.
> products to aid digestion:
>> bile salts to emulsify fats (chenodeoxycholic acid)
>> lecithin to help make cholesterol soluble
>> inorganic salts, including bicarbonate to neutralise duodenal contents.
> at this stage it can go down a number of routes.
  1 Goes into the bile and thus into the small intestine.
  2 Conjugated bilirubin metabolised by colonic bacteria to urobilinogen then stercobilinogen and finally stercobilin (brown colour of faeces).
  3 Some of the urobilinogen is reabsorbed and excreted in the urine.

What are the components of bile?

FRCS candidates have been failed in the past for not being able to answer this. Don't fail for not knowing the basics. Other basic questions that have been asked include: what is albumin?, what is glycogen? and what is the dose of lignocaine?

The main components of bile are:

➤ water
➤ cholesterol
➤ bile pigments
➤ bile acids
➤ phospholipids
➤ bicarbonate.

What are the features of portal hypertension and its consequences?

➤ A portal pressure gradient of >5 mmHg (difference in pressure between the portal and hepatic veins).
➤ Pre-hepatic causes:
  ➢ portal vein thrombosis.
➤ Hepatic causes:
  ➢ cirrhosis
  ➢ hepatic metastasis.
➤ Post-hepatic causes:
  ➢ Budd–Chiari sydrome (thrombosis of hepatic veins).

Complications

➤ Splenomegaly:
  ➢ sequestration of platelets
  ➢ leukopenia, thrombocytopenia – hypertrophy of splendid substance.
➤ Ascites:
  ➢ albumin intravascular oncotic pressure
  ➢ lymph flow through thoracic duct exceeds capacity
  ➢ aldosterone Na and H_2O retention.
➤ Portosystemic shunting varices:
  ➢ gastric, oesophageal
  ➢ periumbilical
  ➢ retroperitoneal
  ➢ rectal
  ➢ diaphragmatic.

LIVER FUNCTION TESTS (LFTs)

➤ Alanine transaminase (ALT):
  ➢ an enzyme present in hepatocytes
  ➢ cell damage leaks it into the blood

➤ raised in acute liver damage, e.g. viral hepatitis or paracetamol overdose.
➤ Aspartate transaminase (AST):
  ➤ enzyme associated with liver parenchymal cells.
  ➤ not specific to the liver, also present in red blood cells and cardiac and skeletal muscle.

The ratio of AST to ALT is sometimes useful in differentiating between causes of liver damage.
➤ Alkaline phosphatase (ALP):
  ➤ enzyme in the cells lining the biliary ducts of the liver
  ➤ rise with large bile duct obstruction, intrahepatic cholestasis or infiltrative diseases of the liver
  ➤ also present in bone.
➤ Total bilirubin:
  ➤ breakdown product of haem (a part of haemoglobin in red blood cells)
  ➤ the liver is responsible for clearing the blood of bilirubin.
➤ Coagulation test (e.g. INR):
  ➤ the liver is responsible for the production of coagulation factors
  ➤ only increased if the liver is so damaged that synthesis of vitamin K-dependent coagulation factors has been impaired.
➤ Serum glucose:
  ➤ gluconeogenesis is the last function to be lost in the setting of fulminant liver failure.
➤ Lactate dehydrogenase (LDH):
  ➤ enzyme found in many body tissues, including the liver. Elevated levels may indicate liver damage.
➤ Gamma glutamyl transpeptidase (GGT):
  ➤ specific to the liver
  ➤ more sensitive marker for cholestatic damage than ALP
  ➤ may be elevated with even minor liver dysfunction
  ➤ raised in alcohol toxicity (acute and chronic).

How would you investigate a patient with jaundice?

The initial management is based around four questions:
➤ What type of jaundice?
➤ What is the cause?
➤ Is it acute or chronic?
➤ Is liver failure present?

Pre-hepatic jaundice
➤ Due to an increased rate of haemolysis, e.g.:
  ➤ malaria
  ➤ sickle-cell anemia

➤ spherocytosis
➤ glucose-6-phosphate dehydrogenase deficiency.
▶ Laboratory findings include:
➤ urine: no bilirubin present
➤ serum: increased unconjugated/indirect bilirubin.

Hepatic jaundice
▶ Cell necrosis reduces the liver's ability to metabolise and excrete bilirubin, e.g.:
➤ acute hepatitis
➤ hepatotoxicity
➤ alcoholic liver disease
➤ congenital disorders.
▶ Laboratory findings include:
➤ urine: conjugated bilirubin present.

Post-hepatic jaundice
▶ Leads to obstructive jaundice as there is blockage of bile flow, e.g.:
➤ gallstones in the common bile duct
➤ pancreatic cancer in the head of the pancreas.

Symptoms include:
➤ presence of pale stools
➤ dark urine
➤ pruritus.
▶ History
▶ Examination
➤ LFTs and other blood tests (see below)
➤ ultrasound in ALL cases
➤ CT/MRI
➤ liver biopsy if no cause identified over 6–12 months.
▶ Specific bloods:
➤ HBsAg – hepatitis B
➤ anti-HCV – hepatitis C
➤ ANA – autoimmune hepatitis
➤ ferritin – haemochromatosis
➤ copper – Wilson's disease.

What is Mirizzi's syndrome
Mirizzi's syndrome (MS) was first described in 1948. PL Mirizzi described an unusual presentation of gallstones, when lodged in either the cystic duct or Hartmann's pouch causing extrinsic compression of the common hepatic duct (CHD) leading to obstructive jaundice.

It comprises four components:
1   Parallel course of the cystic duct to the CHD.

2 Impaction of stones in the cystic duct or neck of the gallbladder.
3 Mechanical obstruction of the CHD by the stones or secondary inflammation
4 Intermittent or constant jaundice and recurrent cholangitis.

Mirizzi's syndrome occurs in about 1% of all patients with cholelithiasis. It is more common in the elderly and has an equal male-to-female distribution. It often escapes detection due to its intermittent symptoms and the limitations of radiological imaging. In MS, the distorted biliary anatomy and marked scarring of the subhepatic space around Calot's triangle, makes surgery difficult and with a significant risk of biliary complications, especially in undiagnosed or unsuspected cases.

McSherry et al. (1982) proposed a classification of MS into Type 1, with external compression of the CHD by a calculus impacted in the cystic duct; and Type 2, where the calculus had eroded into the bile duct creating a cholecystocholedochal fistula. Csendes et al. (1989), in a series of 219 patients, had further sub-classified McSherry Type 2 MS into Type II to IV:

Type 1: No fistula (extrinsic compression only).
Type 2: Cholecystocholedochal fistula (defect <33% diameter CBD).
Type 3: Defect 33–66% CBD diameter.
Type 4: Defect >66% CBD diameter.

Management options

Some authors consider preoperative diagnosis essential in avoiding CBD injuries. Others have concluded that with a cautious intraoperative approach to periductal inflammation and judicious dissection, it is not necessary for successful management. Additional imaging is often needed to obtain details of the biliary pathology because of lack of sensitivity of US and CT scans in discerning the underlying pathology. The most frequently used modality was ERCP. The possibility of stone retrieval and biliary stenting during ERCP is an added advantage in improving surgical outcome, and stenting also facilitates identification of the CBD during operative dissection. However, ERCP is limited by failure to canulate the CBD in 5–10% of cases and suboptimal study from incomplete contrast filling of the ducts due to tight strictures or intraductal debris. Complications including sepsis and pancreatitis can occur after ERCP. When ERCP is unsuccessful or difficult, percutaneous transhepatic cholangiography (PTC) is a viable alternative.

In MS, MRCP can be as good as ERCP in diagnosis and its ability to delineate details of biliary strictures and to detect a cholecystocholedochal fistula. In addition, T2 weighted sections can differentiate a neoplastic mass from an inflammatory one, which US or CT scans may not be capable of. We prefer early ERCP when biliary sepsis is the dominant clinical issue and where a beneficial endoscopic therapeutic procedure can be instituted at the same time. By contrast, MRCP is used to corroborate the suspicion of malignancy after initial imaging with US or CT scans. The dense inflammatory adhesions in Calot's triangle in MS, as well as the frequent aberrant biliary anatomy, pose a difficult challenge to the unsuspecting surgeon when dealing with an MS. Meticulous dissection and vigilance for a potential MS are essential in order to avoid inadvertent bile duct injury. We outline our surgical approach with reference to the literature.

Surgical management

Our surgical strategy aims at tackling the two difficult problems when faced with MS: first, the safe completion of the cholecystectomy without inflicting injury to the bile duct; second, the appropriate management of the cholecystocholedochal fistula. During cholecystectomy, the fundus first approach is favoured over the conventional Calot's first dissection. In acute cholecystitis or when the gallbladder is distended and tense, decompressing it can facilitate dissection. A cholangiogram should be done at this point to confirm the diagnosis, to assess the location and size of the fistula, as well as to exclude the presence of stones or strictures in the bile duct. In a Type 1 MS, the minimum necessary surgery (a cholecystectomy) is adequate. In the absence of CBD stones on pre- or per-operative cholangiogram, stones impacted in the cystic duct or the neck of the gallbladder are milked back into the gallbladder, which is then removed and the cystic duct oversewn. However, the cystic duct is frequently occluded and obscured by inflammatory changes in the region of Calot's triangle. In these cases, a subtotal cholecystectomy, fundus first dissection and leaving the neck of the gallbladder behind, is a more prudent approach. Routine CBD exploration is not necessary unless stones are noted preoperatively or on IOC. Common bile duct exploration should be carried out only if the CBD is easily exposed, otherwise definitive management of CBD stones or stenosis should be left till the inflammatory process has resolved and the situation is reassessed. Bile duct stenosis generally resolves as inflammation subsides following cholecystectomy.

Surgical procedures for Type 2 MS depend on the severity of the fistula and any associated bile duct strictures. A small fistula may be closed primarily by interrupted stitches and a larger defect can be closed using a cuff of gallbladder remnant following subtotal cholecystectomy. Siting of the T-tube following closure of the fistula remains contentious. While some advocate placement through the fistula opening, others suggest that the T-tube be placed through a separate choledochotomy distal to the fistula. It has been advocated for routine biliary bypass of the choledochal fistula to the duodenum or jejunal loop. In a Type IV fistula, where there is complete section of the CHD and questionable vascularity of the CHD, Roux-en-Y hepaticojejunostomy is the procedure of choice. Although all the technical steps necessary in the management of MS are feasible laparoscopically the latter in MS is contentious.

Conclusion

Preoperative diagnosis of MS, especially Type 2, is often inconclusive despite advances in imaging techniques. A high index of suspicion must be maintained when operating on patients with gallstones presenting with a history of jaundice. With meticulous dissection at Calot's triangle and hepatoduodenal ligament as well as adopting the fundus-first approach to the gallbladder, iatrogenic injury and further damage to the bile duct can be avoided.

HEPATOCELLULAR CARCINOMA (HCC)
What are the current guidelines on the management of HCC?
Introduction

There has been much recent debate about the value of surveillance/screening in the diagnosis and management of hepatocellular carcinoma. Rather than recapitulate the arguments that have been aired at length elsewhere, a summary of a proposed methodology for Scotland is described below. It is clear from recent data that the single most effective means that we have impacting on the prognosis of hepatocellular carcinoma is the identification of cases early enough to satisfy criteria for resectional surgery or transplantation. Currently, the majority of patients referred with HCC are unsuitable for curative therapy.

Proposed means of surveillance:
- ➤ ultrasound scan of liver every 6 months in identified high-risk groups (listed below)
- ➤ six-monthly measurement of alpha-fetoprotein. This should be undertaken but will only be used as supporting evidence for image-based diagnoses.

NB: The ultrasound scan should be undertaken by dedicated ultrasonographer (either by a radiologist or radiographer). The distinction between neoplastic nodules and nodular regeneration/macronodular cirrhosis can be extremely difficult and it is recommended that a single dedicated individual undertakes these lists where possible with the 'at risk' patients.

Ideally, clinical nurse specialists associated with cancer services are the most appropriate individuals to call patients for surveillance and screen the initial results, identifying concerning ones for review by medical staff. We recommend that each network work towards the appointment of a specialist nurse to co-ordinate the investigation and treatment of potential/suspected HCC. A similar mechanism should be established for the results to feed directly back to the consultant with responsibility for the patient. Where possible a 'surveillance clinic', which may be a combination of a virtual and actual clinic, should be established and run by a specialist nurse. This would avoid delay in referral after an investigation has highlighted a possible diagnosis of hepatoma.

Estimated burden

Currently, there are established surveillance clinics in Scotland, in Aberdeen

(ARI) and Glasgow (GGH and GRI), which are nurse led. In other locations, surveillance is often undertaken within consultant-led liver or gastroenterology clinics.

High-risk surveillance groups

Patients with chronic hepatitis B/chronic hepatitis B carriers:

➤ Asian males >40 years.

➤ Asian females >50 years.

➤ All cirrhotic hepatitis B carriers.

➤ Family history of HCC.

➤ All African hepatitis B carriers >20 years.

➤ There is an argument for surveying all non-cirrhotic chronic hepatitis B carriers not included in the above. This recommendation is particularly pertinent for patients with high HBV DNA concentrations and those with ongoing hepatic inflammatory activity, as these are at highest risk and should also be screened regardless of age.

➤ All patients with hepatitis B, HIV co-infection, hepatitis C and hepatitis B co-infection should be screened.

Non-hepatitis B cirrhotics:

➤ Hepatitis C.

➤ Alcoholic cirrhotics (surveillance should be undertaken in all patients who are able/willing to cooperate with surveillance and management. Treatment decision should be influenced only by evidence of active drinking).

➤ Haemochromatosis.

➤ Primary biliary cirrhosis (evidence stronger for males than females).

➤ Alpha-1-antitrypsin deficiency.

➤ Non-alcoholic steatohepatitis.

➤ Autoimmune hepatitis. (Evidence for value of surveillance is lacking in this group but if surveillance clinics established then the relatively small numbers with this condition should probably be surveyed if only to provide more substantive data on the relative risk of hepatoma development in this condition. Additionally, we do see hepatoma in patients with 'overlap' syndrome.)

Surveillance of patients post antiviral treatment

This area is still contentious for both hepatitis B and hepatitis C, although studies suggest that the risk of HCC is reduced by interferon or other antiviral drug treatment. On the basis of current evidence and reviews it is suggested that patients with cirrhosis who have been treated with antivirals, whether successful or not (in terms of sero-conversion) should probably continue to be surveyed. This policy can be reviewed if and when clear evidence emerges.

➤ Surveillance should also be undertaken on those patients satisfying criteria and who are on a transplant waiting list.

Diagnosis of HCC

Introduction and setting for diagnostic investigational management

The development of a nodule with abnormal texture in the liver of a patient in the surveillance programme, or identified following de novo investigation, should prompt referral to a hepatologist and urgent further investigation using specialist/experienced radiology/histopathology services. As described below the presence and severity of underlying liver disease impinges on the interpretation of diagnostic tests and the decision to transplant, resect or undertake non-surgical interventions. For these reasons it is suggested that patients are referred via the regional hepatology services (Aberdeen, Dundee, Edinburgh, Glasgow [GRI/GGH/SGH], Inverness) that link with the SLTU and regularly 'fast track' patients to SLTU. It is essential that patients are discussed at the local MDT in the regional hospital in the first instance to triage eligibility for treatment with: transplantation, resection or loco-regional treatment. Where appropriate, patients will be referred to SLTU to define optimal management, assess for transplantation, assess for resectability, to advise on loco-regional treatment E; or enrolment in a clinical should be strongly encouraged where appropriate trials. Patients who should be referred to SLTU include those who satisfy transplant criteria, who are borderline or whom the referring clinician believes may benefit from transplant or review at the SLTU.

Summary of diagnostic approach to suspicious nodules

A viable algorithm for further investigation of such a mass is given in Appendix 1 (adapted from Bruix *et al.*'s *AASLD Guidelines on Management of Hepatocellular Carcinoma*).

Diagnosis is imaging/biopsy based. Although alpha-fetaprotein measurements are used as corroborating criteria to obviate the need for biopsy they play no direct role in the primary diagnosis of HCC.

Proposed recommendations for diagnosis

➤ Lesions >2 cm in diameter and radiological appearance of mass is 'classical' for HCC by confirmatory dynamic modality (CT, MRI), diagnosis can be made 'confidently' (>95% surety) without recourse to biopsy. (If AFP >200, useful as corroborating marker of presence of HCC.)

➤ For large lesions >2 cm without a raised alpha-fetaprotein, current best practice is that two imaging modalities demonstrating classical appearances need to be deployed to obviate the need for a biopsy.

➤ Lesions >2 cm: If appearances are not classical after two dynamic modalities, or there are clinical concerns, or if the lesion is detached in a non-cirrhotic liver, biopsy should be considered. This decision should only be made after work up by hepatologist, hepatobiliary radiologist and hepatobiliary surgeon and follow discussion at the relevant MDT.

Diagnostic modalities may include:

➤ Dynamic diagnostic modalities are: ultrasound scan with contrast, triphasic CT and MRI (+ resovist/gadolinium).

➤ For lesions 1–2 cm diameter that also have 'classical appearances', regardless of alpha-fetoprotein level, two imaging modalities need to be deployed and must demonstrate typical appearances of HCC for diagnosis to be made in absence of biopsy. If diagnostic concern remains then biopsy should be considered after discussion at the relevant MDT as described above.

➤ For lesions <2 cm diameter that do not demonstrate classical appearances on dynamic scanning or that demonstrate a classical appearance on only one imaging modality, a biopsy should be undertaken. If the biopsy is not diagnostic or non-specific, lesion should continue to be monitored (see below).

➤ Lesions <1 cm in diameter: these may be investigated with dynamic imaging. These lesions can be very difficult to separate from regenerative nodules.

➤ Even if these (<1 cm) lesions show a classic 'vascular pattern' it is suggested that the appropriate management should be to repeat the ultrasound/CT at 3-monthly intervals and determine whether these nodules are enlarging. Nodules showing evidence of enlargement should then be managed (more actively) as described above. If the nodules are static or regressive then the patient can re-enter a 6-monthly surveillance programme. NB: In the context of regenerative nodules such as hepatitis B and hepatitis C, alpha-fetoprotein may be raised to a level of above 100IU.

➤ There are a number of caveats about the biopsy of small lesion both relating to targeting the lesion and the pathological interpretation. This needs to be borne in mind when these patients are reviewed at MDT. Expert hepatic pathological input is essential to the diagnosis of these patients. See comments on negative or equivocal biopsy results above. The process of the secondary radiological and histological examination of these patients should take place on a centralised basis.

The role of alpha-fetoprotein measurement

Management should be primarily directed by the identification and characterisation of nodules on imaging, as described above. Nevertheless, alpha-fetoprotein is not entirely redundant in the management of HCC. As described above, alpha-fetoprotein may be raised in association with regenerative activity. A very high alpha-fetoprotein (>200) is strongly indicative of a hepatocellular carcinoma particularly in the context of an isolated nodule >2 cm diameter. In addition, regardless of the absolute level, a relentlessly rising alpha-fetoprotein on serial measurements is concerning and should prompt a vigorous and thorough radiological investigation.

Proposed recommendations for management of HCC
Introduction and setting

➤ Management of hepatocellular carcinoma should take place at a
specialised centre that can offer the multidisciplinary expertise required.
Initial management decisions should be undertaken at the regional
MDT with discussion/referral to SLTU as appropriate (especially if
resection/transplantation is a possible option). Additionally, indications
are changing all the time and this management approach will ensure
patients are treated according to the most up-to-date protocols. The
regional centre should be able to take a multidisciplinary approach
to the diagnosis and management of HCC. Surgeons, anaesthetists,
physicians, oncologists, pathologists and radiologists are required
to inform the management of HCC. This is because the majority
of patients will have significant underlying liver disease creating
anaesthetic and surgical difficulties. Moreover, different approaches to
management are required depending on the stage of the tumour and
clinical status of the patient.

A viable algorithm for management of HCC is given in Appendix 2 (taken
from Bruix *et al.*'s *AASLD Guidelines on Management of Hepatocellular Cancer*).

➤ The prognosis and management of patients with HCC is dependent on
involves the tumour stage/size, the underlying liver function and the
physical status of the patient. Prognostic models including the Okuda
staging and BCLC system give a guide to the underlying outlook; copies
of these are appended (Appendix 3).

➤ A further argument for management in a specialist centre is that
compared to other common tumours, hepatocellular cancer is
hopelessly understudied in terms of controlled trials and particularly
RCTs. Management of patients at specialist centres will facilitate the
design and execution of studies and trials required to answer critical
questions about the natural history and effectiveness of specific
interventions. It will also facilitate the inclusion of patients in phase II
clinical trials of novel therapies.

Specific therapeutic approaches
Surgical resection

Size is less important than topographic position in the liver. Suitability for
resection in those with pre-existing liver disease is determined on the basis
of the Childs-Pugh grading. Patients generally tolerate resection adequately
when they have either:

➤ no cirrhosis (e.g. fibrolomelar HCC) or for patients with underlying
liver disease, those graded Childs-Pugh Grade A or selected Childs
B with an excellent physical performance status and a good quality of
life; or

➤ hepatic vein pressure gradient has also been used as a guide to surgery and it is recommended that this should not exceed 10 mmHg.

Liver transplantation in those unsuitable for resection

Liver transplantation should be considered in all suitable patients, modified Milan criteria should be applied and based on the largest measured parameter of the lesion by CT and/or MRI:

➤ Solitary tumours <5 cm or up to five tumours <3 cm. Absence of nodal spread, vascular invasion, distal spread – requires more intensive and extensive imaging. Absence of significant comorbid factors or other conditions that would impact on suitability for transplantation.

➤ A solitary tumour 5–7 cm that has been stable for 6 months (<20% change in size, AFP <10000) with no new nodule formation, tumour rupture or evidence of vascular invasion.

➤ Patients satisfying these criteria should be referred to SLTU as a matter of urgency for assessment.

Alternative treatments for those unsuitable for resection or OLT

The most appropriate treatment for unresectable HCC has yet to be determined and frequently intervention is offered on the basis of local availability. All patients should be considered for entry into clinical trials. For patients not eligible for entry into trials, treatment is best determined on a multidisciplinary basis at the tertiary referral centre and comprises:

➤ Percutaneous ablation either by RFA or ethanol injection – these approaches work best for small tumours. This means that the significant numbers of patients with large or asymmetric diffuse infiltrating tumours are not suited for this approach. Theoretically this approach in the small well-demarcated tumour can be curative. Setting: specialist/tertiary centres.

➤ Transarterial embolisation and chemo-embolisation (TACE): TACE represents the first-line non-curative therapy for patients unsuitable for resection, transplantation or percuateous ablation. Assessment of portal vein patency is required. Setting: specialist/tertiary centres.

Palliative treatment including chemotherapy

➤ The standard single-agent chemotherapy is doxorubicin 60 mg/kg IV 3-weekly for up to eight cycles, but the response rate is only 20%. The SHARP trial of other approaches are currently being trialled, including the oral multikinase inhibitor sorafenib, which has demonstrated improved survival versus placebo in chemonaive patients with advanced disease. It has not been approved for use in the UK. Recent data with this drug suggests it has a role in compensated cirrhotics that are not candidates for other treatment strategies. However, further data on this is awaited.

➤ Treatments that have been subjected to trials and for which there is no objective evidence to support efficacy should not be deployed. These include:

> tamoxifen
> simvastatin
> anti-androgens
> octreotide
> hepatic artery ligation/embolisation.

➤ Poor performance status, evidence of disseminated disease with extrahepatic spread, evidence of portal vein or hepatic artery compromise, evidence of hyperbilirubinaemia or advanced liver disease, presence of comorbid factors, either in terms of diseases of other systems or other complications associated with liver disease likely to shorten life, may affect suitability for the above treatments and influence 'decision to treat' in these patients. For these patients whose life expectancy is very short, optimisation of symptom control and palliative/symptomatic treatment alone is appropriate. Setting: Local DGH/GP/Community.

➤ Deviation from established protocol should be documented in case records and be made known to the patient's GP. The reason for such deviation should be stated.

PANCREATIC CARCINOMA

What do you know about the aetiology and epidemiology of pancreatic cancer?

Pancreatic cancer is a devastating disease, the seventh leading cause of cancer-related deaths in Ireland, and has one of the lowest 5-year survival rates of any malignancy. Worldwide, approximately 170 000 new cases of pancreatic cancer occur every year. The median survival is 8–12 months for patients presenting with locally advanced and unresectable disease, and only 3–6 months for those with metastatic disease at presentation.

The risk of this malignancy is increased threefold by diabetes. Other factors such as pancreatitis, pernicious anaemia, cystic fibrosis and familial adenomatous polyposis increase the risk of contracting the disease. Cigarette smoking is the only known clear risk factor associated with pancreatic cancer. Cigarette smoking increases the risk of developing pancreatic cancer two- to threefold.

Surgery offers the best possibilities for survival, however only 10% of patients are eligible for resection at the time of diagnosis. Even after resection with curative intent, the 5-year survival rate is approximately 10% ('rule of 10s').

How would you investigate?

Investigations:
➤ carbohydrate antigen (CA 19–9)
➤ ultrasound
➤ triple-phase CT (IV and oral contrast)
➤ ERCP – useful for insertion of stent in context of jaundice and tissue diagnosis

> MRI to seek extent of local invasion
> endoscopic ultrasound (EUS +/– biopsy)
> staging laparoscopy.

Treatment of advanced disease

Gemcitabine is the first-line chemotherapy treatment for pancreatic cancer. This agent is a synthetic nucleoside analogue of the antimetabolite family.

Adding Avastin (bevacizumab) to a combination of Tarceva (erlotinib) significantly improves the time patients with metastatic pancreatic cancer live without their disease getting worse (progression-free survival; PFS).

The result of the phase III AVITA study showed that the addition of Avastin to a Tarceva/gemcitabine combination resulted in:

> a 37% increase in PFS compared to a Tarceva/gemcitabine alone
> almost 14% of patients experiencing a complete regression
> a trend towards improved overall survival.

What are the options for surgical palliation?

> ECRP and stent.
> PTC.
> Choledocho-jenunostomy.
> Choledocho-duodenostomy.
> Hepatico-jejunostomy.

SPHINCTER OF ODDI (SOD) DYSFUNCTION
What is Sphincter of Oddi dysfunction?

Type 1: Biliary pain + deranged LFTs + dilated CBD.
Type 2: Billiary pain + one of the above.
Type 3: Biliary pain only.

What are the principles of management?

The CBD may be dilated on ultrasound >6 mm but this may be up to 9 mm post cholecystectomy. Sphincter of Oddi mamometry (SOM) at ERCP is the gold standard with a normal baseline pressure >40 mmHg. Hepatobiliary scintigraphy (HIDA) scan may show delayed biliary emptying.

The management options are:

> biliary sphincterotomy at ERCP, although this is not ideal for Type 3 patients
> pancreatic stent
> do a cholecystectomy if any evidence of gallstones or sludge on ultrasound.

GALLBLADDER CANCER AND GALLBLADDER POLYPS
What do you know about gallbladder cancer?

Gallbladder cancer is rare with an overall 5-year survival of 5% and a median survival of less than 6 months. The highest incidence of gallbladder cancer is found in indigenous cultures of the Andes Mountains of South America, northeastern Europeans and Israelis. Women are approximately three times more likely to develop gallbladder cancer than men. The most common cited risk factor for the development of gallbladder cancer is gallstones, particularly large stones and cholesterol stones. Other risks are gallbladder polyps >1 cm, and the 'porcelain' gallbladder. This ultrasound finding is an independent risk factor for malignancy and 25% of cases are associated with an underlying malignancy. This finding should be followed with prophylactic cholecystectomy.

Gallbladder polyps

It is generally recommended that a cholecystectomy is performed for any polyp greater than 1 cm, or if the patient is symptomatic. Ultrasound is the diagnostic modality of choice to measure and characterise gallbladder polyps, but if there is any suspicion of malignancy, cross-sectional imaging with contrast-enhanced CT or MRI is essential.

Patients with polyps less than 1 cm who are asymptomatic should be followed initially at 6-monthly intervals to rule out the possibility of a growing adenomatous polyp. The reasons for this policy are several: the overall low risk of malignancy, the fact that simple cholecystectomy is curative for T1 tumours. Prophylactic cholecystectomy for gallstones to prevent gallbladder cancer is not justified.

Incidental finding

An incidental finding of a gallbladder cancer is found in 1 in every 100 laparoscopic cholecystectomies.

The exam question is: You have just taken out an elective gallbladder and the pathology report has just landed on your desk. What will you do next?

The exam answer is:
➤ The case is referred to an HPB surgeon.
➤ The pathology is discussed at an HPB MDT meeting.
➤ The patient has staging investigations, usually CT of the chest and abdomen.

T1 tumours

T1 lesions are usually found incidentally at lap chole pathology specimens and by definition are confined to the mucosa layer and do not penetrate the muscular layer. Cholecystectomy should be curative. It is important that the cystic duct margins are clear.

T2 tumours

These will require liver resection of segment 4 and 5 with regional lymphadenectomy.

T3 tumours

T3 lesions are locally advanced and may be candidates for resection but are likely to have metastatic disease. In general, patients with lymph node disease outside the hepatoduodenal ligament should not undergo hepatic resection.

Describe the aetiology of gallstones

What are the complications of gallstones?
➤ Obstructive jaundice.
➤ Acute pancreatitis.
➤ Biliary colic.
➤ Empyema.
➤ Perforated GB.
➤ Gallstone ileus.
➤ Mirizzi's syndrome.

How do you consent for a laparoscopic cholecystectomy?
Key points:
➤ general and specific complications
➤ conversion to open procedure (5–7%)
➤ DVT
➤ bile duct injury and rates (1 in 400).

What are the key principles of day surgery?
➤ Aim is for 75% of all elective day surgery to be done as a day-case by 2005.
➤ In North America, day-case is defined as patients discharged within 24 hours.
➤ Governed by the British association of day surgery (BADS).
➤ Patients pre-assessed and ready for surgery on arrival.
➤ Separate day-case unit.
➤ Dedicated DCU staff, theatre and ward.
➤ Type of surgery.
➤ Discharge criteria.
➤ Protocols and guidelines.
➤ Staged patient recovery.
➤ Nurse-led preassessment clinic.
➤ GPs to have direct access to minor ops.
➤ Audit.
➤ Follow-up on request.

How do you establish a pneumoperitoneum?

Two options:
> ➤ Veress technique
> ➤ open Hasson cut-down.

Both are essentially now justified and appropriate. Make a choice on your preferred technique, perfect it, taylor it to your operation and stand behind your decision in the exam.

What are the complications of laparoscopic surgery?

The wide acceptance of laparoscopic surgery is due to the advantages of early recuperation, reduced pain, shorter hospitalisation, improved cosmesis, and lower morbidity and mortality compared with the open procedure. The possible complications of laparoscopic surgery can be divided into the following complications.

Laparoscopy-related complications
> ➤ Visceral injuries.
> ➤ Vascular injuries.
> ➤ Trocar site injury.
> ➤ Hypothermia.
> ➤ Acidosis.
> ➤ Raised ICP.
> ➤ V/Q mismatch.
> ➤ Arrhythmias.
> ➤ Hypotension.
> ➤ Bradycardia.
> ➤ Reduced cardiac output.
> ➤ Oliguria.

Visceral injuries are uncommon, occurring in 0.05–0.4% of all laparoscopic procedures. The most common offender is the veress needle and visceral injury is the most common cause of late morbidity and mortality due to laparoscopic access. These patients typically present with peritonitis 2–7 days after surgery.

Regarding vascular injuries, the indications for laparotomy and formal vascular repair are an expanding retroperitoneal haematoma, haemodynamic instability or active intra-abdominal haemorrhage. Mortality due to retroperitoneal injury secondary to trocar insertion ranges from 9–36%.

Pneumoperitoneum, long operating time and the reverse Trendelenburg position predispose the patient to DVT. Gas embolism may occur with intravascular insufflations. It presents with sudden hypotension, cardiac arrhythmias and decreased cardiac output. The treatment is to release the pneumoperitoneum, place the patient in the Durant position (i.e. head down on the left lateral position), insert a central line and aspirate the air embolism from the right ventricle.

The haemodynamic cardiovascular effects are typically seen at the start of the procedure. Decreased cardiac output, hypotension, and bradycardia are typical. These patients should have adequate preoperative volume loading together with pneumatic compression stockings for the lower limbs. Both the head-up position and the elevated intra-abdominal pressure independently reduce venous return to the heart.

The induction of a CO_2 pneumoperitoneum may cause hypercapnia and lead to a respiratory acidosis. The head-down position may reduce lung compliance and lead to ventilation/perfusion (V/Q) mismatch. Lowering the intra-abdominal pressure and controlling the ventilation rate reduced the respiratory acidosis during pneumoperitoneum.

Patient-related complications
➤ Urinary retention.
➤ Ileus.
➤ Aspiration pneumonia.
➤ Adhesions.
➤ Pregnancy.

Surgery-specific complications
Laparoscopic cholecystectomy:
➤ bile duct injury (1 in 200, 0.5%).

TEP/TAPP:
➤ hernia recurrence
➤ neuralgia
➤ bleeding
➤ ischaemic orchitis
➤ retroperitoneal haematoma.

Laparoscopic fundoplication:
➤ perforation of stomach
➤ pneumothorax
➤ oesophageal perforation
➤ bleeding
➤ liver injury
➤ splenic injury.

What are the key points of the NICE guidelines for laparoscopic repair of inguinal hernias?
The evidence is based on 37 randomised controlled trials (RCTs) involving up to 5500 patients including various meta-analyses.

Key points
➤ Laparoscopic repair is the preferred method of repair for both bilateral and recurrent hernias.
➤ It is an option for primary unilateral hernia.
➤ It appears to be cost-effective.
➤ The TEP repair is 7.8 minutes longer than the open repair.
➤ Return to work is 3 days sooner with TEP repair.
➤ TEP has less pain at 1 year.
➤ Recurrence rate is similar with TEP versus open.
➤ TAPP causes more vascular/visceral injuries.
➤ TEP causes less pain post-op.
➤ TEP causes less numbness post-op.

ACUTE CHOLECYSTITIS
Which antibiotic(s) do you use for acute cholecystitis?
➤ Gram-negative aerobes (50%).
➤ *Enterococcus* (30%).
➤ Anaerobes (15%).
➤ Ceftrixone/gentamycin + flagyl.
➤ Ceftrixone and metronidazole IV (www.bsac.org.uk).

What do you know about single port cholecystectomy?

Laparoscopic cholecystectomy remains the most frequently performed minimally invasive operation for general surgeons. The next step toward 'scar-less' surgery uses a modified single multichannel port inserted through the umbilicus.

The use of a single port requires modification of the currently established technique for laparoscopic cholecystectomy with a single-port protocol. This new method presents a few technical difficulties and challenges compared with the conventional 3-port or 4-port laparoscopic cholecystectomy.

Results from an Aberdeen study of 30 patients (all females) with no intra-operative/postoperative complications, conducted from September 2008 to March 2009 showed 20 of 30 patients had their operation completed with the use of a single port. An extra 5 mm epigastric port was required in 8 of the 20 patients. Another 2 out of 20 patients required conversion of the operation into a standard laparoscopic technique (one 3-port and one 4-port procedure). All the patients were discharged within 24 hours. There were no intraoperative or postoperative complications or mortalities.

The single-port technique is feasible for performing routine laparoscopic procedures. With further advances in surgical technique, technology and instrumentation, this technique can be reproduced to perform more complex biliary and other procedures in future.

What do you think about day-case lap chole?

Day-case laparoscopic cholecystectomy (LC) is a viable option for certain patients. A randomised clinical trial of day-case versus overnight stay published in the *British Journal of Surgery* confirmed this (Parvaiz and Hafeez; 2006). The main features of the trial were:

➤ Department of Surgery, University Hospital, Sweden
➤ 100 patients
➤ aged 18–70 years
➤ ASA I-II
➤ exclude if CBD stone, acute cholecystitis, pancreatitis, >50 km
➤ randomised to day-case or overnight stay
➤ n = 52 vs n = 48.

Results

➤ 48 (92%) home within 4–8 hours post-op.
➤ No patient was re-admitted.
➤ 2% conversion rate.
➤ Reduction in cost (€3085 vs €3394).

When do you operate in acute cholecystitis?

Early cholecystectomy is now considered the correct mode of treatment in otherwise fit patients and is backed up by a 2006 Cochrane review. The main results were as follows, with no significant differences between most primary outcomes.

The Cochrane review was backed up by a large meta-analysis of 12 RCTs. The implications for clinical practice are:

➤ early LC during acute cholecystitis safe
➤ shortens hospital stay
➤ CBD stones are important issue
➤ only 20% surgeons in the UK perform LC during acute cholecystitis (Senapati 2003)
➤ LC within 72 hours (ideally 48 hours)
➤ day-case procedure possible for electives.

How common are bile duct injuries?

Regarding prevention and risk factors:

➤ 70% of surgeons regard bile duct injuries as unavoidable
➤ most occur during first 100 LCs
➤ one-third occur after surgeons' first 200
➤ misidentification of anatomy is the commonest cause of injury (70–80%)
➤ no RCT on effect of IOC with incidence of bile duct injury.

When are bile duct injuries more likely to occur?

➤ Varied anatomy.

➤ Obesity.
➤ Inadequate exposure.
➤ Poor clip placement.
➤ Diathermy near CBD.
➤ Acute cholecystitis.
➤ Inexperience of surgeon
➤ Cystic duct and CBD aligned in same plane (excessive cephalic traction).
➤ Chronic inflammation.
➤ Impacted stone in Hartmann's pouch.

How are you going to diagnose it?
➤ 90% of injuries are not diagnosed during surgery.
➤ High index of suspicion required.
➤ Patient unwell at 48 hours post-op.
➤ Jaundice, sepsis, biliary peritonitis.
➤ Bloods (FBC, LFTs, amylase, clotting).
➤ Ultrasound is initial investigation.
➤ Laparoscopy if peritonitis present.

What would be your first-line radiological investigation?
➤ Ultrasound.
➤ Look for residual CBD stones.
➤ Biliary dialation.
➤ Fluid collection.

If jaundiced post lap chole or CBD dilated, then patient needs urgent ERCP/ stent.

All cystic duct stump leaks resolved by ERCP.

What is your management strategy for common bile duct (CBD) stones?
Option 1: If ultrasound confirms dilated CBD = ERCP + sphincerotomy.
Option 2: Laparoscopic CBD exploration.
Option 3: If the above fails, then open CBD exploration +/– T-tube.

A 55-year-old man is jaundiced on the first post-op day following lap chole. How do you proceed?
Any patient presenting with jaundice immediately post lap chole should have an urgent ERCP. Bile duct injury must be assumed till proven otherwise. The exam scenario will be along the lines of either jaundice post lap chole or another scenario in which the patient becomes unwell on the first post-operative day following an apparently straight forward operation. Examiners may differ in the management here. You must be confident in what YOUR management will be here.

The two common scenarios are:

➤ Bile leak with subsequent biloma/biliary peritonitis: in this case the patient will be unwell on the first postoperative day with pyrexia and raised WCC together with localised peritonitis. What I have been taught to do here is to put the laparoscope back in. **Do re-laparoscopy first.**

➤ Total occlusion of CBD causing obstructive jaundice: this patient will need an ERCP. The most likely injury will be that the clips have come off the cystic duct and this can be remedied with a stent.

How would you manage a liver abscess?

➤ Image
➤ Radiological guidance
➤ Microbiology

THE SPLEEN
How do you classify splenic trauma?

How would you do an emergency splenectomy for trauma?

➤ Midline.
➤ Four-quadrant packing.
➤ With LEFT hand spleen mobilised to midline.
➤ Splenic ligamentous attachments are divided with scissors or diathermy to allow for rotation of the spleen to midline.
➤ Identify the splenic artery and vein for ligation.
➤ Once the splenic artery and vein are identified and controlled by ligation.
➤ The gastrosplenic ligament with the short gastric vessels is divided and ligated near the spleen to avoid injury or late necrosis of the gastric wall.
➤ Drains are typically unnecessary unless concern exists over injury to the tail of the pancreas during operation.

What are the complications of a splenectomy?

➤ Recurrent splenic bed bleeding (24–48 hours).
➤ Pancreatitis/pancreatic fistula/pseudocyst.
➤ Gastric necrosis/perforation.

➤ Subphrenic collections/abscess.
➤ OPSI (5% lifetime risk).
➤ DVT (thrombocytosis/platelets).
➤ Portal vein thrombosis (get contrast CT).
➤ Acute gastric dialatation.

What are the main principles of managing overwhelming postsplenectomy infection (OPSI)?
➤ 5% lifetime risk in splenectomy patients.
➤ Higher in children.
➤ Highest risk within 2 years post-op.
➤ Lifelong risk remains.
➤ Pneumonia or meningitis in half the cases.
➤ Vaccines (Hib, Pneumovax, Meningovax).
➤ Oral penicillin V 250 mg BD.
➤ *Strep. pneumoniae* accounts for 90% OPSI.
➤ Mortality up to 60%.

ACUTE PANCREATITIS
What are the causes of pancreatitis?
➤ Gallstones.
➤ Ethanol.
➤ Trauma.
➤ Steroids.
➤ Mumps.
➤ Autoimmune.
➤ Hypercalcaemia, hyperlipidaemia.
➤ Drugs (AZT, valproate).

Other pancreatitis facts
➤ 3% of all cases of abdominal pain in UK.
➤ Overall mortality 10–15%.
➤ One-third die in early phase from MOF.
➤ Necrotising pancreatitis mortality 40%.
➤ Amylase diagnostic at three times the normal limit.
➤ Serum lipase diagnostic at twice the normal limit.

What is serum lipase?
➤ Elevated serum amylase and lipase levels in combination with abdominal pain trigger the initial diagnosis of acute pancreatitis.
➤ Serum lipase rises 4–8 hours from the onset of symptoms and normalises within 7–14 days after treatment. If the lipase level is about 2–3 times that of amylase, it is an indication that alcohol is the aetiological factor.
➤ Serum amylase may be normal (in 10% of cases) for cases of acute or chronic pancreatitis due to depleted acinar cell mass.

Regarding selection on these tests, two practice guidelines state:

It is usually not necessary to measure both amylase and lipase. Serum lipase may be preferable because it remains normal in some nonpancreatic conditions that increase the amylase level. In general, serum lipase is thought to be more sensitive and specific than serum amylase in the diagnosis of acute pancreatitis.

Although amylase is widely available and provides acceptable accuracy of diagnosis, where lipase is available it is preferred for the diagnosis of acute pancreatitis (recommendation Grade A).

How do you assess disease severity in acute pancreatitis?

What are the complications of pancreatitis?

What is the CT severity index of Balthazar (CTSI)?

CTSI score is from 0 to 10 and is composed of the CT grading of the pancreatitis 0–4 plus the necrosis score 0–6.

CT score
0   Normal
1   Pancreatic enlargement
2   Peri-pancreatic inflammation
3   Extensive fluid collection
4   Multiple abscess

Necrosis score
0   None
2   30%
4   50%
6   >50%

What is the role of antibiotics in acute pancreatitis?

You should have a definite plan of when and where you will use antibiotics in pancreatitis and have some evidence to back it up. This is an area of controversy and that is just what the examiners like.

A 2008 Cochrane review based on five meta-analyses looking at prophylaxis of infection of pancreatic necrosis concluded a trend to decreased mortality with no increased risk of fungal infection. It supports the use of proven necrosis on CT and advocated using a 2-week course of either imipenum or meropenum. Nationally, there is no support for routine use in all cases of pancreatitis and the BSG have no specific recommendations.

When do you image in pancreatitis?

➤ CT (contrast enhanced) 6–10 days.
➤ Contrast-enhanced CT vs MRI.
➤ Necrosis CT = MRI.
➤ Fluid collection MRI > CT.

What are the indications for necrosectomy?

Gas on CT
➤ Indicates infected necrosis.
➤ Necrosectomy indicated (40% mortality).

Positive FNA culture
➤ Necrosectomy indicated.

What is the evidence for percutaneous pancreatic necrosectomy?

According to 2003 NICE guidelines, the current evidence does not support the use of percutaneous necrosectomy. The mortality rates range from 0–25%. The specialist advisory committee has commented that the use of the above may cause exacerbation of existing sepsis, incomplete clearance of necrosis and recurrence.

The risk of fistula formation has ranged from 15–25%. The conversion to laparotomy is up to 33% and so should not be performed outside specialist centres with registry facilities.

What is the role for ERCP in acute pancreatitis?

According to BSG guidelines:
➤ all cases of pancreatitis of gallstone aetiology
➤ bilirubin >90
➤ dilated CBD on ultrasound.

Ideally, an early ERCP (i.e. within 72 hours) should be performed. There are three RCTs that show a reduced mortality.

What are the complications of an ERCP and how would you manage them?

➤ Bleeding
➤ Perforation
➤ Pancreatitis

How would you investigate a case of pancreatitis with no gallstones and no alcohol?

➤ First, repeat the ultrasound by a good radiologist.
➤ Check bloods for calcium, triglycerides and auto-antibodies.
➤ Exclude drugs.
➤ EUS/ERCP.
➤ CT scan to exclude malignancy.

Only 10% of cases should be attributed to being idiopathic.

BENIGN LIVER LESIONS

A common exam question is to be given an ultrasound report with a liver lesion and then you must explain how you, as a consultant, will manage the patient. There are five main lesions you will get.

1 Haemangioma.
2 Liver cell adenoma.
3 Focal nodular hyperplasia.
4 Simple cyst.
5 Cystadenoma.

Haemangioma

➤ This is the commonest benign liver lesion.
➤ It does not undergo malignant change.
➤ Most are asymptomatic till >10 cm.
➤ Intra-abdominal rupture is rare.
➤ Typical patients are young females.
➤ The most important point is that ultrasound CANNOT distinguish between a haemangioma, HCC, liver cell ademona, FNH or a solitary liver metastasis and so a CT is required, at least, for diagnosis.

Liver cell adenoma

➤ These usually occur in young females.
➤ They are related to pregnancy and the OCP usage

➤ 10% are associated with a risk of rupture.
➤ 10% will have a risk of malignant transformation.
➤ Formal liver resection is required for symptomatic patients.

Focal nodular hyperplasia (FNH)
➤ FNH is a benign process.
➤ It is not pre-malignant.

Simple cyst
➤ Symptomatic cysts can be deroofed laparoscopically.

Cystadenoma
➤ These are rare.
➤ There is malignant potential.
➤ They grow very slowly.
➤ Complications include: biliary obstruction, haemorrhage, sepsis and malignancy.
➤ In view of the risk of malignant transformation into cystadenocarcinoma, a cystadenoma of the liver, even if asymptomatic, MUST be treated by complete excision.

What are the anatomical variations of the cystic artery?
In approximately 70% of cases, the cystic artery originates from the right hepatic artery. When the superficial and deep branches of the cystic artery do not share a common origin it is defined as a double cystic artery occurring with a frequency of 15%.

Unusual anatomy of the right hepatic itself can occur with an aberrant branch of the right hepatic artery. This is typically from the SMA and may occur with a frequency of 15%.

Colorectal

> ➤ Bowel preparation
> ➤ Benign anorectal disorders
> ➤ Diverticular disease
> ➤ Inflammatory bowel disease
> ➤ Colorectal cancer
> ➤ Chemotherapy for colon cancer
> ➤ Laparoscopic colorectal surgery

BOWEL PREPARATION
Bowel prep or not?
Downside of bowel prep

Hypovolaemia
- ➤ Decreased cardiac output/shock.
- ➤ Decreased coronary artery perfusion.
- ➤ Collapse.
- ➤ Colonic mucosal ischaemia.

Electrolyte disturbance
- ➤ Fits.
- ➤ Dysrhythmias.
- ➤ Myopathy.
- ➤ Nausea.
- ➤ Diarrhoea.
- ➤ Lack of sleep.

Irving et al. *(1987)*
- ➤ Retrospective, uncontrolled study.
- ➤ No bowel prep.
- ➤ 72 primary anastomoses.

➤ No leaks.
➤ 8% wound sepsis.

What do you know about ERAS?

Enhanced recovery is a programme of multidisciplinary care designed to minimise postoperative organ dysfunction and return the patient to normality as soon as possible.

ASGBI guidelines 2009 summary

➤ Should be a team approach.
➤ Pre-op counselling essential.
➤ Pre-load carbohydrate.
➤ 2 hours to clear liquid pre-op.
➤ No bowel prep.
➤ DVT prophylaxis essential.
➤ Single-dose antibiotics.
➤ 80% FIO2 for at least 6 hours post-op.
➤ Avoid hypothermia.
➤ Goal-directed fluid therapy.
➤ Use of short/transverse incisions.
➤ No drains.
➤ No NG tubes.
➤ Early diet and mobilisation.
➤ Regular unit audit.

Evidence base

➤ Basse (2000).
➤ Post-op hospital stays in 60 patients undergoing elective colonic resection.
➤ 32 out of 60 home within 48 hours.

Wind *et al.* (2006)

➤ One systematic review of all RCTs and controlled trials on fast-track colonic surgery.
➤ Six papers analysed.
➤ Three RCTs.
➤ N = 512.
➤ Effect of length of stay: overall 1.6 days.
➤ Effect of morbidity: decrease 50%.
➤ Readmission rate not statistically significant.
➤ No increase in mortality.

Practical points

➤ Pre-operative counselling.
➤ Selective/no bowel prep.

➤ Carbohydrate loading.
➤ Stimulation of gut motility.
➤ Vertical nursing.
➤ Thoracic epidurals.
➤ Smaller incisions.
➤ No drains.
➤ No pre-med.
➤ Euvolaemic fluid replacement.
➤ Drip down day 1.
➤ Ignore urine output.
➤ Daily creatinine.
➤ Urine 0.3 mL/kg/hr.
➤ BP 90 systolic.
➤ No NG tubes.
➤ Home day 3.
➤ Audit results.

BENIGN ANORECTAL DISORDERS
How do you manage faecal incontinence?
Common causes of faecal incontince

➤ Trauma:
  ➢ obstetric
  ➢ surgical
  ➢ accidental.
➤ Colorectal disease:
  ➢ haemorrhoids
  ➢ prolapse
  ➢ IBD
  ➢ tumours
  ➢ resections.

Examination

➤ Full examination including neurological.
➤ Perineum:
  ➢ strain to assess perineal descent and exclude prolapse
  ➢ inspection: previous surgery, conditions
  ➢ closed or patulous anus
  ➢ PR: resting tone, squeeze pressure; rectocele
  ➢ sigmoidoscopy + proctoscopy.

Structural assessment

➤ Endoscopic ultrasound (EUS):
  ➢ accurately identifies internal and external sphincter defects
  ➢ useful for deciding upon surgery.

➤ 3D EUS will improve accuracy, also better imaging of supporting structures.
➤ Endoanal MRI:
  ➣ more sensitive for external sphincter
  ➣ atrophy identified by fatty infiltration
  ➣ led to realisation puborectalis atrophy important
  ➣ useful for identifying those for surgery.

Treatment
➤ Loperamide:
  ➣ synthetic opioid and Ca blocker
  ➣ increases fluid reabsorption and reduces secretions
  ➣ affects sphincter and increases resting tone
  ➣ more effective than any other agent
  ➣ use syrup to titrate dose
  ➣ safe and no tolerance.
➤ Phenylephrine cream:
  ➣ alpha-1-adrenergic agonist
  ➣ increases resting tone (needs intact sphincter)
  ➣ contact dermatitis a problem.

Biofeedback
➤ Re-conditioning pelvic floor.
➤ Visual or auditory feedback to encourage sphincter synchrony and strength.
➤ Feedback by manometry, EMG or EUS.
➤ Combined with sensory feedback using balloon distension.
➤ Reduce panic.
➤ Rectal retrograde irrigation.
➤ Adjuvant hypnotherapy may help.
➤ Cures half and improves two-thirds.

Surgical options
➤ Post anal repair:
  ➣ restore 'anorectal angle'
  ➣ posterior plication of levator and external sphincter
  ➣ radiology fails to show association between function and improvement
  ➣ has fallen out of favour
  ➣ less than one-quarter continent at 6 years.
➤ SECCA procedure:
  ➣ allied to STRETTA for GORD
  ➣ radiofrequency energy delivered to muscularis
  ➣ fibrosis and scarring
  ➣ bleeding, ulceration, pain
  ➣ 60 patients at 2 years 'modest or better improvement'.

What are the guidelines for sacral nerve stimulation?

Sacral nerve stimulation:
➤ NICE approved
➤ few complications
➤ shown to improve QoL
➤ 75–100% improved
➤ 41–75% completely continent
➤ maintained at 2 years (only procedure)
➤ indications: mixed sphincter injuries, spinal injuries, sphincter defects.

Current evidence on the safety and efficacy of sacral nerve stimulation for faecal incontinence appears adequate to support the use of this procedure, provided that the normal arrangements are in place for consent, audit and clinical governance.

The procedure should only be performed in specialist units by clinicians with a particular interest in the assessment and treatment of faecal incontinence.

In patients for whom conservative treatments have been unsuccessful, surgical alternatives include tightening the sphincter (overlapping sphincteroplasty), creating a new sphincter from the patient's own muscle (for example, dynamic graciloplasty) or implanting an artificial sphincter. Some patients may require colostomy. Sacral nerve stimulation is a surgical treatment option for patients with faecal incontinence.

Commonly, the procedure is tested in each patient over a 2- to 3-week period, with a temporary percutaneous peripheral nerve electrode attached to an external stimulator.

If significant benefit is achieved, then the permanent implantable pulse generator can be implanted.

How do you manage anal fissures?

➤ 90% of all anal fissures will heal spontaneously without surgery.
➤ ACPGBI position statement advocates topical diltiazem 2% BD for 6 weeks.

What is your technique for lateral sphincterotomy?

➤ Lithotomy position.
➤ Eisenhammer retractor.
➤ Palpation of IAS.
➤ Local with adrenaline.

➤ 11-blade scalpel.
➤ Division of 25% of muscle.

What is the evidence for Botox in anal fissure?

Compared with placebo, we don't know whether botulinum A toxin–haemagglutinin complex is more effective than placebo at reducing the proportion of people with anal fissure at 2 months (low-quality evidence).

Compared with topical glyceryl trinitrate, we don't know whether botulinum A toxin-haemagglutinin complex is more effective than topical glyceryl trinitrate at reducing the proportion of people with anal fissure at 2 months (low-quality evidence).

Compared with nifedipine, we don't know whether botulinum A toxin-haemagglutinin complex is more effective than nifedipine at reducing the proportion of people with anal fissure at 30 days (low-quality evidence).

Compared with internal anal sphincterotomy botulinum A toxin-haemagglutinin complex is less effective than internal anal sphincterotomy at reducing the proportion of people with anal fissure at 6–12 months (high-quality evidence).

What are surgical options for repairing a pilonidal sinus?

Systematic review and meta-analyses of randomised controlled trials have been conducted looking into outcomes of time (days) to healing, surgical site infection and recurrence rate. Secondary outcomes were time to return to work, other complications and morbidity, cost, length of hospital stay and wound healing rate. 18 trials (n = 1573) were included. 12 trials compared open healing with primary closure. Time to healing was quicker after primary closure although data were unsuitable for aggregation. Rates of surgical site infection did not differ; recurrence was less likely to occur after open healing (relative risk 0.42, 0.26 to 0.66). Fourteen patients would require their wound to heal by open healing to prevent one recurrence. Six trials compared surgical closure methods (midline vs off-midline). Wounds took longer to heal after midline closure than after off-midline closure (mean difference 5.4 days, 95% confidence interval 2.3 to 8.5), rate of infection was higher (relative risk 4.70, 95% confidence interval 1.93 to 11.45), and risk of recurrence higher (Peto odds ratio 4.95, 95% confidence interval 2.18 to 11.24). Nine patients would need to be treated by an off-midline procedure to prevent one surgical site infection and 11 would need to be treated to prevent one recurrence.

In summary, wounds heal more quickly after primary closure than after open healing but at the expense of increased risk of recurrence. Benefits were clearly shown with off-midline closure compared with midline closure.

Off-midline closure should become standard management for pilonidal sinus when closure is the desired surgical option.

Discuss how you would perform an EUA for acute peri-anal sepsis?
➤ Identify external opening(s).
➤ Perineal palpation to assess track:
  ➢ not palpable = not intersphincteric.
➤ PR (anal) any indentation or induration. Ask patient to squeeze to help locate external sphincter and puborectalis.
➤ PR (rectal) any induration (feels like bone).
➤ DRE by colorectal surgeon 85% accurate.

Summary
➤ Drain the pus.
➤ Do not meddle.
➤ Document the relation to the pigmented skin.
➤ Document the relation to the clock face.
➤ History if intermittent pain building to passage of pus – fistula likely.
➤ Bacteriology 100% sensitive and 60–80% specific.
➤ Prospective trial of 200 cases anal sepsis:
  ➢ simple drainage vs primary fistulotomy
  ➢ recurrence: 36.7% vs 5%
  ➢ complications: 0% vs 2.8%.
➤ EUA:
  ➢ downward traction of dentate may aid identification of openings
  ➢ Eisenhammer traction may reveal a dimple
  ➢ massage of tract may reveal pus
  ➢ instil saline, hydrogen peroxide or dyes
  ➢ gentle probe.
➤ Hx, Ex, proctosigmoidoscopy.
➤ Essential five points:
  1 Location of internal opening.
  2 Location of external opening.
  3 Course of primary track.
  4 Presence of secondary extensions.
  5 Presence of other complicating diseases.

What is a fistula-in-ano?
Defined as a track or cavity communicating with the rectum or anal canal by an identifiable internal opening.

Aetiology
➤ 90% idiopathic.
➤ 10%:

➤ Crohn's disease
➤ hidradenitis
➤ TB
➤ malignancy.

How do you classify fistula-in-ano?

Classification

➤ Intersphincteric (45%): Usually simple, though may be complicated.
➤ Transsphincteric (29%): Track passes through external sphincter into ischiorectal fossa.
➤ Suprasphincteric (20%): Run up above puborectalis then curl down through levators and ischiorectal fossa.
➤ Extrasphincteric (5%): Not related to sphincters.

Problems

➤ Superficial fistulas out with this classification.
➤ Difficult to clinically differentiate, e.g. intersphicteric and low transsphincteric.
➤ Suprasphincteric not cryptogladular.
➤ Some argue that suprasphincteric fistula doesn't exist.
➤ Primary track.
➤ Internal opening.
➤ External opening.
➤ Secondary extensions or abscesses.

What is Goodsall's rule?

Goodsall's rule states that with the patient in the lithotomy position and an imaginary horizontal line drawn through the anus, where the external opening of the fistula is above the line the fistula tract will extend radially, and where the external opening is below the line then the tract will open in the midline.

What are the principles of surgery for fistula-in-ano?

➤ Drain acute sepsis.
➤ Aim to treat chronic tracks.
➤ Secondary tracks should be laid open, curetted or drained.
➤ Antibiotic cover if complex.
➤ Debate about bowel prep.
➤ Lithotomy or prone.

What are the options for managing a 50-year-old female with rectal prolapse?

➤ Image large bowel and exclude other pathology.
➤ Assess fitness for surgery.
➤ Discuss options for surgery:

➤ Delorme's
➤ Altemeire's
➤ Resection rectopexy
➤ Open/laparoscopic.

How do you treat haemorrhoids (piles)?
➤ Haemorrhoids contribute to continence.
➤ Haemorrhoids worth preserving.
➤ Haemorrhoids are graded from 1 to 4.
➤ Grade 1: bleeding.
➤ Grades 2–4: prolapse.
➤ Most do not require surgery.
➤ Avoid banding at outpatient clinic.

DIVERTICULAR DISEASE
How do you classify diverticular disease?
➤ Hinchey I: pericolic abscess confined to mesentery of colon.
➤ Hinchey II: walled off pelvic abscess.
➤ Hinchey III: generalised peritonitis.
➤ Hinchey IV: faecal peritonitis.

How would you manage a 70-year-old man with acute diverticulitis?
Key points
➤ Sigmoid diverticular disease is common.
➤ Emergency admission is uncommon.
➤ Contrast CT is ideal investigation.
➤ Urgent surgery in <25% of cases.
➤ Abscess <5 cm resolve with IVABs.
➤ Sigmoid resection is best option with primary anastomosis in selected cases.

When would you operate in diverticular disease?
➤ Free air under diaphragm.
➤ Generalised peritonitis.
➤ Progressive signs and failure of medical Rx after 3 days in hospital.

How do you do a Hartmann's procedure?
➤ Lloyd-Davies position.
➤ Midline.
➤ Mobilise splenic flexure.
➤ Rectal stump suture and washout.
➤ IVABs for 3–5 days.
➤ Reversal possible in 50% cases.

INFLAMMATORY BOWEL DISEASE
Describe the medical management of IBD

The ASCEND I and II clinical trials evaluated overall treatment success as the primary endpoint. The pooled results from ASCEND I and II showed that moderate UC patients who were treated with mesalazine (Asacol) 800 mg M/R at 4.8 g/day had more rapid symptom relief in terms of blood in the stool and stool frequency than patients who received 2.4 g/day.

The median time to symptom relief was 10 days faster for those on the higher dose ($p = 0.02$). The patients receiving the higher dose also experienced a higher rate of treatment success at 6 weeks.

Oral 5-ASA

➤ 5-ASA are effective in the induction and maintenance of remission in UC Grade A).
➤ ASCEND II found that 4.8 g/day is better than 2.4 g/day in treating moderately active UC.
➤ 4 g/day no more effective in preventing recurrence than 1.2 g/day.
➤ Adherence to therapy is vital to emphasise as a fivefold increase in relapse rate when compliance <80%.
➤ Adding topical 5-ASA to oral 5-ASA therapy can also help in frequently relapsing disease.
➤ Regular 5-ASA may reduce risk of colorectal cancer in patients with UC.
➤ A case-control study found that 5-ASA use reduced CRC risk by 81%.
➤ Regular hospital visits also reduced risk.
➤ A family history of sporadic CRC increased risk fivefold.
➤ May help with patient compliance.

Steroids

➤ Remain standard therapy for inducing remission in moderate/severe UC (Grade A).
➤ Trials conducted over 40 years ago.
➤ No evidence to support their use in maintenance of remission (Grade A).
➤ No benefit from more than 40 mg.

Azathioprine

➤ Until recently, relatively weak Grade C evidence.
➤ The azathioprine-withdrawal study provided stronger evidence (Grade A).
➤ 53% vs 21% in remission and steroid free at 6/12 when compared to 5-ASA.

Cyclosporine

➤ No RCT data.
➤ Use based on the Lichtiger study where 75% short-term response in severe UC.
➤ At best, 55% avoid surgery at 3 years.

➤ Significant side-effect profile.
➤ Lower dose, 2 mg/kg may be better tolerated.

Biological therapy

Turning to biological therapy, the ACT I and II trials demonstrated that Infliximab effectively induced clinical responses in patients with moderate to severe UC that was active despite conventional therapy.

➤ ACT I and II have demonstrated its efficacy in the induction and maintenance of remission in UC (Rutgeerts *et al.* 2005).
➤ Significantly better than placebo in inducing and maintaining remission in moderate to severe UC.
➤ Significantly more treated patients were able to achieve steroid-free remission.
➤ Improved quality of life scores.
➤ Also studied as a single infusion as rescue therapy in acute severe UC.
➤ Significantly fewer patients in the Infliximab-treated group had a colectomy (29% vs 67%).
➤ No serious side-effects.
➤ Cost £2000 per infusion.

How would you manage a 28-year-old with acute toxic megacolon?

➤ The Oxford study (1988) demonstrated that at day 3 of IV hydrocortisone, if
  ➢ BO × 8/day or
  ➢ BO × 3–8 with CRP >45 mg/l
➤ 85% would require colectomy.

If >3 stools (with blood) a day at day 7, there was a 60% chance of continuous symptoms and 40% chance of colectomy.

What are the complications of pouch surgery?

➤ Procedure associated with 30% morbidity.
➤ Pouch failure.
➤ Pelvic sepsis (20%).
➤ Poor function (20%).
➤ Pouchitis (10%).
➤ Pouch-vaginal fistula (5–10%).
➤ SBO, PE, DVT, bleeding, infection, wound complications.

A good pouch has a patient with 5–6 bowel motions per day and 1–2 per night. The single ONLY advantage is that the patient avoids a stoma.

What are the principles of managing intestinal failure?

Intestinal failure is defined as the inability to maintain adequate nutritional, fluid and electrolyte status without supportive therapy. The main causes in adults are Crohn's disease and short bowel syndrome.

There are three stages:
➤ high output/hypersecretion phase
➤ adaptation phase
➤ stabilisation phase.

The principles of management of an enteral fistula are listed by SNAP.

Sepsis
➤ Resuscitate.
➤ Establish reliable venous access.
➤ Correct electrolyte imbalance.
➤ Correct Hb to optimal level.
➤ Identify and control sepsis (drainage +/– antibiotics).

Nutrition
➤ Restrict oral fluid to 500 mL/day.
➤ Start H2 antagonists/proton-pump inhibitors.
➤ Loperamide prn (ac).
➤ Octreotide 100 mg s/c TDS.
➤ Diorylte with added sodium.
➤ Oral magnesium supplements.
➤ <1500 mL losses may be controlled with oral replacement alone.
➤ >2000 mL will require TPN.

Anatomy
➤ Define the extent of disease.
➤ Exclude distal obstruction.
➤ Delineate the fistula tract and the level of the fistula.
➤ Exclude sepsis/intra-abdominal collections.

Procedure
➤ En-bloc resection.
➤ Primary anastomosis.

How does the management of a post-op fistula differ from a spontaneous enterocutaneous fistula?

Post-op fistula
➤ Wait at least 6 weeks. A post-op fistula will heal in around 70% cases, usually within the first 6 weeks of starting TPN.
➤ They are usually entero-cutaneous.
➤ They will usually close with conservative management.

Spontaneous fistula
- ➤ These will not heal spontaneously.
- ➤ Patients tend to be less symptomatic.
- ➤ Bowel perforation tends to be more slowly.
- ➤ There are benefits from early surgery as there is usually no previous surgery.

COLORECTAL CANCER
How would you stage rectal cancer?
Treatment decisions should be made with reference to the TNM classification. The American Joint Committee on Cancer (AJCC) has designated staging by TNM classification and recommended that at least 12 lymph nodes be examined in patients with colon and rectal cancer to confirm the abscence of nodal involvement by tumour.

What is downstaging?
Downstaging is reducing the T-stage of a large tumour with long-course chemoradiotherapy.

What do you know about the CR07 trial?
The CR07 trial was a British Medical Research Trial (MRC) published in 2006. It was a randomised trial to assess whether local recurrence-free rates were different by giving short course preoperative radiotherapy, or to give postoperative chemo-radiotherapy only to those at high risk of recurrence.

A total of 1350 patients were randomised, as this was the number required to detect a 2.5% difference at 5% significance with 90% power. The primary end-point of local recurrence at 3 years was 4.7% for pre-op and 11.1% for post-op groups.

Therefore, short course preoperative radiotherapy resulted in a significantly reduced rate of local recurrence and improved disease-free survival at 3 and 5 years when compared with the highly selective postoperative group.

What is HNPCC?
Hereditary non-polyposis colorectal cancer (HNPCC) was previously known as Lynch syndrome and is a genetic cause of colorectal cancer. It is responsible for about 2% of colorectal cancers and is inherited in an autosomal dominant fashion. For diagnosis they should either fit the Amsterdam criteria or have been genetically tested and demonstrated to have microsatelite instability (MSI) and defective mismatch repair gene (MMR). The risk of colorectal cancer is 80% (compared with a 100% risk of colonic cancer in FAP).

Management
- ➤ Annual colonoscopy from age 25 to 75.

➤ There is no evidence that a patient with a family history should have a prophylactic colectomy.
➤ Annual OGD from age 50 to 75.

Surgical options
➤ Colectomy and ileorectal (rectal surveillance).
➤ Segmental resection (and continued surveillance).
➤ Total colectomy and IPAA.

Risk of cancer is 3% per annum in the retained rectum.

Genes implicated in HNPCC
➤ MLH1 (90% of cases).
➤ MSH2 (90% of cases).
➤ MSH6 (10% of cases).
➤ PMS.
➤ PMS2.

Microsatellites are repeated sequences of DNA. The appearance of abnormally long or short microsatellites in an individual's DNA is called microsatellite instability (MSI). MSI is a condition manifested by damaged DNA due to defects in the normal DNA repair process.

What do you know about the Amsterdam criteria?
The Amsterdam criteria are criteria in identifying high-risk candidates for molecular genetic testing for HNPCC.

Amsterdam criteria (1990)
➤ Three or more family members with a confirmed diagnosis of colorectal cancer, one of whom is a first-degree relative of the other two (parent, child, sibling).
➤ Two successive generations affected.
➤ One or more colon cancers diagnosed under 50 years of age.
➤ FAP has been excluded.

Amsterdam criteria (1999)
➤ Three or more family members with HNPCC-related cancer, one of whom is a first-degree relative of the other two.
➤ Two successive affected generations.
➤ One or more of the HNPCC-related cancers diagnosed under 50 years of age.
➤ FAP has been excluded.

What is FAP?
➤ Risk of colorectal cancer in those with FAP approximates 100%.

> Mutation of tumour suppressor adenomatous polyposis coli (APC) gene C5q.
> Autosomal dominant inheritance.
> Polyp dense and attenuated forms.
> Characterised by hundreds of adenomas at a young age.
> Gastroduodenal adenomas.
> Extraintestinal manifestations: epidermoid cysts, CNS tumours, desmoid tumours, bony lesions, Ca duodenum, stomach, SB, thyroid, adrenal, biliary tract.

What is a TME?
> Total mesorectal excision or else mesorectal excision to 5 cm distal to the lower extent of the tumour.
> Preservation of hypogastric nerves.
> Anterior and antero-lateral dissection around Denonvilliers' fascia in males is critical.

What nerves may be damaged in TME?
The superior third of the rectum is covered by peritoneum over its anterior and lateral surfaces. The Total Mesorectal Excision (TME) is the surgical plane between the fascia propria of the rectum and the parietal fascia. The mesorectum is an extension inferiorly from the mesosigmoid. It contains the terminal and proximal branches of the IMA and IMV and lymphatics glands.

The pre-sacral fascia covers the sacral nerves and vessles. The anococygeal ligament splits to form Waldeyer's fascia to reach the anorectal junction where it joins the fascia propria of the rectum. The superior portion of the pre-sacral fascia contains the superior hypogastric nerve plexus.

The lateral ligaments are a thickening of the lateral connective tissues of the rectum. They contain the middle rectal artery and rectal branches of the superior hypogastric plexus.

The superior hypogastric plexus (sympathetic) L5
The SHN runs laterally along the pelvic wall behind the parietal fascia. The left branch is situated behind the Superior Rectal Artery (SRA). Inferiorly, the SHN trunks extend towards the posterior lateral edges of the seminal vesicles where anterior afferent branches supply the anterior pelvic organs. On the medial aspect, the SHN gives branches directly to the rectum via the lateral ligaments.

Inferior hypogastric plexus
These receive supply from superior hypogastric plexus and S2, S3, S4. The external anal sphincter is supplied by S2, S3, S4, via the pudendal nerve. All these run deep to the pelvic fascia and travel towards anterior portion of Denonvilliers' fascia. Avoiding dissection anterior to Denonvilliers' fascia therefore protects these nerve branches.

What do you know about anal cancer?

Anal tumours account for about 4% of anorectal malignancies. The majority (80%) are squamous cell in origin (SCC). The anal canal begins where the rectum enters the puborectalis sling and ends at the squamous mucocutaneous junction with the perianal skin. The proximal canal is lined with colonic (columnar epithelium) mucosa. The dentate line is lined with a narrow zone of transitional mucosa. Below this is non-keratinising squamous epithelium between the dentate line and mucocutaneous junction.

The incidence of anal carcinoma is increasing. A peak incidence is noted in the seventh decade, with females more commonly affected than males (5:1). Recognised risk factors include female gender, lifetime number of sexual partners, Crohn's disease, cervical carcinoma, HPV infection, anal intercourse and cigarette smoking.

Bowen's disease refers to squamous carcinoma in-situ in both keratinising and non-keratinising epithelium. The natural history of this condition is unknown. Following confirmation of Bowen's disease the area is widely excised with a 1 cm margin.

Patients typically present with a perianal mass with or without pruritus ani, pain and bleeding.

Endoanal ultrasound (EAUS) is the gold-standard investigation for local staging. It is more accurate than CT for predicting T-stage and nodal status.

Palpable inguinal lymphadenopathy should undergo FNAC.

A large clinical trial has shown that the treatment of choice for anal squamous carcinoma is a combination of radiotherapy and intravenous 5-FU.

How do you manage AIN?

Anal intra-epithelial neoplasia (AIN) is a pre-malignant condition, the natural history of which is unknown. It is graded I–III.

Grade I and II run a slow and benign course and should be observed at 6-monthly intervals.

Grade III is a high-grade disease and if the lesions are small (<1 cm) they should be excised. Larger lesions should be biopsied regularly at 6-monthly intervals.

A 65-year-old male presents with malignant large bowel obstruction. How would you proceed?

This is a common scenario and you should have a coherent strategy.

Following AXR suspicion of large bowel obstruction a water-soluble gastrograffin enema should be first-line investigation. This will allow you to distinguish between a definite mechanical obstruction and either pseudo-obstruction and/or sigmoid volvulus. The evidence for this is from Koruth and Mathieson (1985).

A 65-year-old male patient admitted with abdominal distension and vomiting. Gastrograffin enema confirms mechanical large bowel obstruction at the recto-sigmoid junction. You proceed to laparotomy. What do you do next?

Surgical options
➤ Synchronous tumour (4%): subtotal colectomy.
➤ Tumour at splenic flexure: extended right-hemicolectomy.
➤ Upper rectal cancer: single-stage procedure.
➤ Unfit and septic patient: Hartmann's.
➤ Healthy bowel: segmental resection.

The evidence for a single-stage procedure comes from the SCOTIA trial (1995) involving 91 patients. This compared sub-total colectomy to segmental resection with on-table lavage. The results showed no difference in mortality or hospital stay. The segmental resection was better in terms of stoma rate and bowel function.

CHEMOTHERAPY
How is adjuvant chemoradiotherapy given?
The following are recommended as options for the adjuvant treatment of patients with stage III (Dukes' C) colon cancer:
➤ capecitabine as monotherapy
➤ oxaliplatin in combination with 5-FU/folinic acid.

In the UK, about 25% of patients diagnosed with colorectal cancer are classified as having stage III (or C1, C2 according to the modified Dukes' score). These patients have an overall 5-year survival rate of between 25% and 60%. After a complete surgical resection, patients with stage III colon cancer have a 50% chance of developing recurrent disease.

After multidisciplinary team (MDT) discussion, adjuvant chemotherapy should be scheduled to begin 6 weeks post-op and the standard treatment is a 6-month course of 5-FU and folinic acid (5-FU/FA) given IV.

Pooled data from clinical trials suggest that 5-FU/FA regimens will increase disease-free survival at 5 years from 42% to 58%, and overall survival from 51% to 64%, when compared with surgery alone.

Capecitabine
Capecitabine (Xeloda) is an orally administered precursor of 5-fluorouracil (5-FU). It is licenced for the adjuvant treatment of patients following surgery of stage III disease and first-line monotherapy for metastatic colorectal cancer. Capecitabine is contraindicated in patients with severe leucopenia, neutropenia, or thrombocytopenia, and in patients with severe hepatic or severe renal impairment. Dose-limiting side-effects are: diarrhoea, stomatitis, and hand and foot syndrome.

Oxaliplatin

Oxaliplatin (Eloxatin) is a platinum-based cytotoxic drug that prevents DNA replication. Peripheral neuropathy may be dose limiting. It is given in combination with 5-FU/FA.

The X-ACT (Xeloda – Adjuvant Chemotherapy) trial investigated the efficacy and safety of capecitabine versus 5-FU/FA in post-op Dukes' C patients. In the long-term follow-up capecitabine was as effective as the IV 5-FU.

The MOSAIC trial (Multicentre International Study of Oxaliplatin/ Fluorouracil/Leucovorin in the Adjuvant Treatment of Colon Cancer) combined oxaliplatin with 5-FU/FA in the 'de Gramont' regimen and compared 5-FU/FA alone. The addition of oxaliplatin led to a statistically significant reduction in rate of relapse when compared to 5-FU alone. In the interim analysis report there was no statistically significant difference in overall survival.

What is the role for palliative chemotherapy for advanced or metastatic colorectal cancer?

A recent Cochrane review (2009) involving 13 RCTs and a total of over 1000 patients demonstrated that palliative chemotherapy was associated with a 35% reduction in risk of death. This translates into an improvement in median survival of 3.7 months.

Chemotherapy is effective in prolonging time to disease progression and survival in patients with advanced colorectal cancer.

LAPAROSCOPIC COLORECTAL SURGERY

What is the evidence for laparoscopic colorectal surgery?

Benefits for laparoscopic surgery

➤ Less bleeding.
➤ Less postoperative pain.
➤ Less complications.
➤ Less postoperative stay.
➤ Earlier return to normal activity.

All the above are obtained with no compromise in leak rate or in oncological clearance.

Trials

The three main trials to know about:
➤ COST (Clinical Outcomes of Surgical Therapy):
   ➤ 870 patients
   ➤ longer operating time
   ➤ quicker recovery and shorter stay
   ➤ no difference in mortality or morbidity
   ➤ no difference in tumour recurrence or survival.

➤ COLOR (Colon Cancer Open or Laparoscopic Resection):
  ➢ conversion rate 17%
  ➢ outcomes similar to COST trial.
➤ CLASSIC (Conventional versus Laproscopic Assisted Surgery In Patients with Colorectal Cancer):
  ➢ UK multicentre trial
  ➢ this trial included rectal cancer
  ➢ 29% conversion rate
  ➢ there was a higher rate of positive circumferential resection margin (CRM) with the laparoscopic group.

Meta-analysis
➤ Functional outcome:
  ➢ minor improvement in early recovery.
➤ Local complications:
  ➢ significant reduction in wound complications.
➤ Recurrence:
  ➢ no difference in local recurrence
  ➢ no difference in wound recurrence (1%)
  ➢ no difference in distant recurrence.

Conclusions from the meta-analysis:
➤ better short-term outcomes without compromise in oncological outcomes
➤ no difference in 3-year survival, disease-free survival or local recurrence
➤ benefits were confirmed in old age
➤ benefits were confirmed in the obese
➤ port site recurrence was similar to open surgery.

Current NICE guidelines suggest that laparoscopic surgery should be offered to patients.

Upper GI

MANAGEMENT OF UPPER GI BLEED
Proton pump inhibitors (PPIs) for acute GI bleed
A 2009 Cochrane review (Leontiadis *et al.* 2010) reviewed 24 RCTs with approx 4000 patients. The results showed there was no difference in all-cause mortality compared to placebo. PPI did reduce rebleeding rate and decreased surgery rate.

BENIGN UPPER GI
H. pylori in non-ulcer dyspepsia
A 2009 Cochrane review (Moayyedi *et al.* 2011) conducted a meta-analysis of 21 RCTs. In 17 of the trials there was no difference at 1 year with NNT = 14. Hence there is a small benefit, so it is probably worth treating.

SIGN guidelines for the management of dyspepsia suggest that this should be investigated after the age of 55 with or without alarm symptoms.

HOW WOULD YOU MANAGE A BLEEDING DUODENAL ULCER?
Acute upper gastrointestinal bleeding
Studies confirm an extremely high fatality in inpatients of 42%. The following factors are associated with a poor outcome, which is defined in terms of severity of bleed, uncontrolled bleeding, rebleeding, need for intervention and mortality. These factors should be taken into account when determining the need for admission or suitability for discharge.
➤ Age: mortality due to UGIB increases with age across all age groups.
➤ Comorbidity: the absence of significant comorbidity is associated with mortality as low as 4%.
➤ Liver disease: cirrhosis is associated with a doubling of mortality and much higher risk of interventions such as endoscopic haemostasis or transfusion.
➤ The overall mortality of patients presenting with varices is 14%.

Inpatients have approximately a threefold increased risk of death compared to patients newly admitted with GI bleeding. This is due to the presence of comorbidities in established inpatients rather than increased severity of bleeding.

Initial shock (hypotension and tachycardia) is associated with increased mortality (OR 3.8) and need for intervention.

There is conflicting evidence on the value of nasogastric aspiration. A bloody aspirate may indicate a high-risk lesion (sensitivity 48%, specificity 76%) but no evidence has been identified that it alters outcome.

Acute lower gastrointestinal bleeding

There is limited evidence available on the initial assessment of patients with acute lower gastrointestinal bleeding.

The available evidence identifies the following factors associated with uncontrolled bleeding and/or death.

➤ Age: acute lower GI bleeding occurs most often in the elderly. The precise relationship between age and mortality is statistically less well defined than for UGIB.
➤ Acute haemodynamic disturbance (OR 3 to 4.3) and gross rectal bleeding on initial examination (OR 2.3 to 3) are important predictors of subsequent severe bleeding.
➤ Comorbidity: the presence of two comorbid conditions doubles the chance of a severe bleed (OR 1.9).
➤ The patient's history is important for accurate assessment of risk and can give important clues to the diagnosis and need for admission. For example, a history of previous LGIB from a known diagnosis of diverticular disease (the commonest cause of LGIB accounts for 23–48% of cases) predicts a further episode with a 10% chance of recurrence at 1 year and 25% at 4 years.
➤ Diverticular bleeds resolve spontaneously in 75% of cases.

Pre-endoscopic risk assessment

Acute upper gastrointestinal bleeding

Simple and widely validated scoring systems to identify patients at high risk of rebleeding, death and active intervention are needed for optimum management.

The Rockall scoring system was principally designed to predict death based on a combination of clinical and endoscopic findings. Given that many of the risk factors for rebleeding are identical to those for mortality and that rebleeding itself is independently predictive of death, the Rockall score may also be used to estimate rebleeding risk.

Rockall score is derived from age (0–2 points), shock (0–2 points) and comorbidity (0–3 points). The minimum score of 0 is assigned to patients under 60 years of age who have no evidence of shock and/or comorbidity. A score of 0 identifies 15% of patients with acute UGIB at presentation who have an extremely low risk of death (0.2%) and rebleeding (0.2%), and who may be suitable for early discharge or non-admission

WHEN WOULD YOU INVESTIGATE GORD?

Stefanidis *et al.* and the SAGES Guidelines Committee (2010) produced the definitive guideline for antireflux surgery.

Definition

The Montreal consensus defined gastroesophageal reflux disease as 'a condition which develops when the reflux of stomach contents causes troublesome symptoms and/or complications'. 'Troublesome' indicating symptoms adversely affect an individual's well-being.

Surgically GORD is the failure of the lower oesophageal pressure gradient created by the diaphragmatic hiatus, allowing abnormal reflux of gastric contents into the oesophagus. It may also be attributed to a gastric emptying disorder, or failed oesophageal peristalsis. Hence there is a wide spectrum of disease and varied persentations. Colloqial 'heartburn' is the most common but this may be difficult to distinguish from advanced disease with underlying tissue damage or even malignancy. The exact components envolved with the creation of the lower oesophageal 'sphincter' are still not completely understood but as well as the diaphragmatic crura the phrenoesophageal ligament is thought to be important.

Diagnosis

Endoscopy should always be the first step in assesment. If endoscopy is normal with no changes attributable to reflux the current gold-standard objective test to diagnose gastroesophageal reflux is the 24-hour ambulatory oesophageal pH-metry. Factors with the highest proven specificity and sensitivity are: total time with pH <4 as recorded by a probe placed 5 cm above the sphincter, and a composite score (comprised of the following six variables: (1) total oesophageal acid exposure time, (2) upright acid exposure time, (3) supine acid exposure time, (4) number of episodes of reflux, (5) number of reflux episodes lasting more than 5 minutes and (6) the duration of the longest reflux episode). There is a 48-hour wireless probe available but as yet no advantage has been confirmed from the longer duration of assessment.

Recommendation

Based on the available evidence, the diagnosis of GORD can be confirmed if at least one of the following conditions exists: a mucosal break seen on endoscopy in a patient with typical symptoms, Barrett's oesophagus on biopsy, a peptic stricture in the absence of malignancy, or positive pH-metry (Grade A).

SAGES Guideline Committee

Indications for surgery

Consider surgery if reflux is confirmed and the patient has:

➤ Failed medical management (inadequate symptom control, severe regurgitation not controlled with acid suppression, or medication side-effects).

OR

➤ Complications of GORD (e.g. Barrett's oesophagus, peptic stricture).

OR

➤ Extra-oesophageal manifestations (asthma, hoarseness, cough, chest pain, aspiration).

OR

➤ Persued surgery despite successful medical management (due to quality of life considerations, lifelong need for medication intake, expense of medications, etc.).

Preoperative investigations

1 OGD.
2 pH-manometry.
3 Oesophageal manometry: may help identify conditions in which fundoplication is contraindicated (i.e. achalasia) or allow objective decisions about type of fundoplicaiton performed.

Medical versus surgical treatment

Seven randomised controlled trials with follow-up ranging from 1 to 10.6 years have compared surgical therapy with medical therapy for the treatment of GORD. They support the use of surgery even if medical therapy controls symptoms (level 1 evidence).

One randomised control study evaluated the cost difference between omeprazole therapy and fundoplication. In Denmark, Norway and Sweden medical therapy was cheaper (but more expensive in Finland).

Recommendation

Surgical therapy for GORD is an equally effective alternative to medical therapy and should be offered to appropriately selected patients by appropriately skilled surgeons (Grade A).

SAGES Guideline committee

Surgical technique, learning curves and their influence on outcome

In order to standardize literature and clarify the long-term outcome of fundoplication it has been suggested that a standardised approach be undertaken

(as designed by a group of 40 experts):
1 Opening of the phrenoesophageal ligament in a left to right fashion.
2 Preservation of the hepatic branch of the anterior vagus nerve.
3 Dissection of both crura.
4 Transhiatal mobilisation to allow approximately 3 cm of intra-abdominal oesophagus.
5 Short gastric vessel division to ensure a tension-free wrap.
6 Crural closure posteriorly with nonabsorbable sutures.
7 Creation of a 1.5–2 cm wrap with the most distal suture incorporating the anterior muscular wall of the oesophagus.
8 Bougie placement at the time of wrap construction.

Laparoscopic versus open treatment of GORD
In the most recent meta-analysis, perioperative morbidity was found to be significantly lower (65%) after laparoscopic compared with open fundoplication.

Predictors of success
Preoperative patient compliance with antireflux medications
Patients who are most compliant with PPI treatment and who have a good response to treatment are most likely to benefit from fundoplication.

Age
Age has not been found to significantly affect the outcomes of antireflux surgery. Age >65 may be associated with >90% success rate.

Psychological disease and intervention
Cognitive behavioural therapy and full assessment may have a role but as yet unclear.

Revisional surgery for failed antireflux procedures
Most authors recommend the same surgical approach for the reoperative patient as for the primary procedure. Multiple retrospective studies have evaluated the short- and long-term outcomes of revisional laparoscopic antireflux surgery with up to 12 years follow-up. Compared with primary repair, revisional surgery requires longer operative times and is associated with higher conversion rates to open surgery (level III), and higher complication rates (30 day mortality <1%, esophagogastric perforations in 11 to 25%, gastric more often than esophageal perforation, pneumothorax in 7% to 18%, splenic injuries in 2%, and vagal nerve injuries in 7%). Nevertheless, postoperative dysphagia (3% to 17%) and gas bloat syndrome (5% to 34%) do not seem to be significantly higher after reoperation compared with primary repair.

Patient satisfaction after reoperative laparoscopic antireflux surgery has been reported to be high (89%) with resolution of heartburn symptoms in 68% to 89% of patients and resolution of regurgitation in 83% to 88% up to

18 months after revisional surgery. Nevertheless, up to 13% of patients may experience reflux recurrence at 3 months follow-up based on objective testing.

Postoperative complications
Complication rates following antireflux surgery vary related to experience, technique, and degree and intensity of follow-up. Conversion rates to open surgery for laparoscopic antireflux surgery range from 0 to 24%; however, series from high-volume centres report conversion rates <2.4%.

Pneumothorax has been reported but it is rare and infrequently requires intervention.

Postoperative use of acid reducing medications
The resumption of acid reducing medications in patients after antireflux surgery has been reported to range widely (0 to 62%) at both short- and long-term follow-up. Long-term medication use has been reported to range from 5.8% to 62% with most studies reporting rates <20%. One randomised controlled trial, however, reported a 62% incidence of antacid medication resumption after antireflux surgery, which constitutes a very high rate compared with the rest of the literature.

HOW DOES A CLO TEST WORK?
Rapid urease test, also known as the CLO test (*Campylobacter*-like organism test), is a rapid test for diagnosis of *Helicobacter pylori*. The basis of the test is the ability of *H. pylori* to secrete the urease enzyme, which catalyses the conversion of urea to ammonia and bicarbonate. The test is performed at the time of gastroscopy. A biopsy of mucosa is taken from the antrum of the stomach, and is placed into a medium containing urea and an indicator such as phenol red. The urease produced by *H. pylori* hydrolyses urea to ammonia, which raises the pH of the medium, and changes the colour of the specimen from yellow (negative) to red (positive). There is evidence to suggest that *H. pylori* moves proximal in the stomach in patients on therapy with proton pump inhibitors, and, as such, samples from the fundus and antrum should be taken in these patients.

TELL ME ABOUT *H. PYLORI*?
H. pylori is a helix-shaped Gram-negative bacterium. Colonisation of the stomach by *H. pylori* results in chronic gastritis, an inflammation of the stomach lining. The severity of the inflammation is probably the cause of *H. pylori*-related diseases. Duodenal and stomach ulcers result when the consequences of inflammation allow the acid and pepsin in the stomach lumen to overwhelm the mechanisms that protect the stomach and duodenal mucosa from these caustic substances. The type of ulcer that develops depends on the location of chronic gastritis, which occurs at the site of *H. pylori* colonisation. The acidity within the stomach lumen affects the colonisation pattern of

H. pylori and therefore ultimately determines whether a duodenal or gastric ulcer will form. In people producing large amounts of acid, *H. pylori* colonises the antrum of the stomach to avoid the acid-secreting parietal cells located in the corpus (main body) of the stomach. The inflammatory response to the bacteria induces G cells in the antrum to secrete the hormone gastrin, which travels through the bloodstream to the corpus. Gastrin stimulates the parietal cells in the corpus to secrete even more acid into the stomach lumen. Chronically increased gastrin levels eventually cause the number of parietal cells to also increase, further escalating the amount of acid secreted. The increased acid load damages the duodenum, and ulceration may eventually result. In contrast, gastric ulcers are often associated with normal or reduced gastric acid production, suggesting that the mechanisms that protect the gastric mucosa are defective. In these patients, *H. pylori* can also colonise the corpus of the stomach, where the acid-secreting parietal cells are located. However, chronic inflammation induced by the bacteria causes further reduction of acid production and, eventually, atrophy of the stomach lining, which may lead to gastric ulcer and increases the risk for stomach cancer.

Diagnosis of infection is usually made by checking for dyspeptic symptoms and by tests that can indicate *H. pylori* infection. One can test noninvasively for *H. pylori* infection with a blood antibody test, stool antigen test or with the carbon urea breath test (in which the patient drinks ^{14}C – or ^{13}C-labelled urea, which the bacterium metabolises, producing labelled carbon dioxide that can be detected in the breath). However, the most reliable method for detecting *H. pylori* infection is a biopsy check during endoscopy with a rapid urease test, histological examination, and microbial culture. There is also a urine ELISA test with a 96% sensitivity and 79% specificity. None of the test methods are completely failsafe. Even biopsy is dependent on the location of the biopsy. Blood antibody tests, for example, range from 76% to 84% sensitivity. Some drugs can affect *H. pylori* urease activity and give false negatives with the urea-based tests.

Treatment

Once *H. pylori* is detected in patients with a peptic ulcer, the normal procedure is to eradicate it and allow the ulcer to heal. The standard first-line therapy is a 1-week 'triple therapy' consisting of proton pump inhibitors such as omeprazole, lansoprazole and the antibiotics clarithromycin and amoxicillin. Variations of the triple therapy have been developed over the years, such as using a different proton pump inhibitor, as with pantoprazole or rabeprazole, or replacing amoxicillin with metronidazole for people who are allergic to penicillin. Such a therapy has revolutionised the treatment of peptic ulcers, and has made a cure to the disease possible; previously, the only option was symptom control using antacids, H_2-antagonist or proton pump inhibitors alone.

H. pylori is contagious, although the exact route of transmission is not known. Person-to-person transmission by either the oral–oral or faecal–oral route is most likely. Consistent with these transmission routes, the bacteria have been isolated from faeces, saliva and dental plaque of some infected people. Transmission occurs mainly within families in developed nations yet can also be acquired from the community in developing countries. *H. pylori* may also be transmitted orally by means of fecal matter through the ingestion of waste-tainted water, so a hygienic environment could help decrease the risk of *H. pylori* infection.

WHAT IS BARRETT'S OESOPHAGUS? (AND WHAT WOULD YOU DO IF YOU FOUND IT?)

Barrett's oesophagus is defined as the columnisation of distal oesophagus by intestinal metaplasia. It is thought to be a precursor to adenocarcinoma.
➤ Long segment: >3 cm length.
➤ Short segment: <3 cm length.

Risk factors:
➤ males
➤ age
➤ extended segment >8 cm
➤ GORD >10 years
➤ family history
➤ obesity
➤ smoking.

The pathology will determine the management.
➤ Intestinal metaplasia: 2-yearly OGD surveillance.
➤ Low-grade dysplasia + PPI and re-biopsy at 3 months. If stable, then biopsy at 6 months.
➤ High-grade dysplasia: repeat the biopsy and the current recommendation is that surgery should be offered if both are positive as up to 40% of high-grade dysplasia will have focus of adenoca. Endoscopic ablation is an alternative in those unfit for surgery.

WHAT ARE GISTs?

Gastrointestinal stromal tumours (GISTs) were previsusly called leiomyomas and are mesenchymal tumours of the GI tract. They develop as well demarcated spherical masses arising out of the muscularis propria. They express tyrosine kinase.

They are usually in the upper GI tract with 70% arising from the stomach. They typically present as GI bleeding (70%) and up to half of cases will require a laparotomy for bleeding.

Surgcial resection is the treatment of choice aiming for an R0 resection. Imatinib mesylate (Glivec) is a tyrosine-kinase inhibitor and can increase survival from 25% to 75% at 2 years.

NICE guidelines recommend imatibin 400 mg daily as first line for CD 117-positive unresectable tumours. This should only be continued if there is a good response to treatment at 3 months. The annual cost of treatment is £19 000.

HOW DO YOU MANAGE ACHALASIA?

Achalasia is an esophageal motility disorder involving the smooth muscle layer of the oesophagus and the lower oesophageal sphincter (LOS). It is characterised by incomplete LOS relaxation, increased LOS tone, and aperistalsis of the oesophagus (inability of smooth muscle to move food down the oesophagus) in the absence of other explanations like cancer or fibrosis.

Achalasia is characterised by difficulty swallowing, regurgitation, and sometimes chest pain. Diagnosis is reached with esophageal manometry and barium swallow. Various treatments are available, although none cure the condition. Certain medications or Botox may be used in some cases, but more permanent relief is brought by esophageal dilatation and surgical cleaving of the muscle (Heller myotomy).

The aetiology of achalasia is, as yet, unclear.

Signs and symptoms

The main symptoms of achalasia are dysphagia (difficulty in swallowing) and regurgitation of undigested food. Dysphagia tends to become progressively worse over time and to involve both fluids and solids. Some achalasia patients also experience weight loss, coughing when lying in a horizontal position, and chest pain which may be perceived as heartburn. The chest pain experienced can often be mistaken for a heart attack. Food and liquid, including saliva, are retained in the oesophagus and may be inhaled into the lungs (aspiration).

Due to the similarity of symptoms, achalasia can be mistaken for more common disorders such as gastroesophageal reflux disease (GORD), hiatus hernia, and even psychosomatic disorders.

Investigations

Lower oesophageal cancer must always be ruled out with an upper gastrointestinal endoscopy. The internal tissue of the oesophagus generally appears normal in endoscopy, although a 'pop' may be observed as the scope is passed through the non-relaxing lower esophageal sphincter with some difficulty, and food debris may be found above the LOS.

Barium swallow

'Bird's beak' appearance is typical in achalasia.

Treatment

Sublingual nifedipine significantly improves outcomes in 75% of people with mild or moderate disease. Surgical myotomy provides greater benefit than either botulinum toxin or dilation in those who fail medical management.

Lifestyle changes
Both before and after treatment, achalasia patients may need to eat slowly, chew very well, drink plenty of water with meals, and avoid eating near bed-time. Raising the head of the bed or sleeping with a wedge pillow promotes emptying of the oesophagus by gravity. After surgery or pneumatic dilatation, proton pump inhibitors can help prevent reflux damage by inhibiting gastric acid secretion; and foods that can aggravate reflux, including ketchup, citrus, chocolate, alcohol, and caffeine, may need to be avoided.

Medication
Drugs that reduce LOS pressure may be useful. These include calcium channel blockers such as nifedipine and nitrates such as isosorbide dinitrate and nitroglycerin. However, many patients experience unpleasant side-effects, such as headache and swollen feet, and these drugs often stop helping after several months.

Botulinum toxin (Botox) may be injected into the lower oesophageal sphincter to paralyse the muscles holding it shut. As in the case of cosmetic Botox, the effect is only temporary and lasts about 6 months. Botox injections cause scarring in the sphincter, which may increase the difficulty of later Heller myotomy. This therapy is only recommended for patients who cannot risk surgery, such as elderly persons in poor health.

Pneumatic dilatation
In balloon (pneumatic) dilation or dilatation, the muscle fibers are stretched and slightly torn by forceful inflation of a balloon placed inside the lower esophageal sphincter. Gastroenterologists who specialise in achalasia and have performed many of these forceful balloon dilatations achieve better results and fewer perforations. There is always a small risk of a perforation that requires immediate surgical repair. Pneumatic dilatation causes some scarring which may increase the difficulty of Heller myotomy if the surgery is needed later. Gastroesophageal reflux occurs after pneumatic dilatation in some patients. Pneumatic dilatation is most effective on the long term in patients over the age of 40; the benefits tend to be shorter-lived in younger patients. It may need to be repeated with larger balloons for maximum effectiveness.

Surgery
Heller myotomy helps 90% of achalasia patients. The myotomy is a length-wise cut along the oesophagus, starting above the LOS and extending down onto the stomach a little way. A partial fundoplication or 'wrap' is generally added in order to prevent excessive reflux, which can cause serious damage to the oesophagus over time. After surgery, patients should keep to a soft diet for several weeks to a month, avoiding foods that can aggravate reflux.

Most recommended fundoplication along with Heller's myotomy is Dor's fundoplication. It consists of 180- to 200-degree anterior wrap around the oesophagus. It provides excellent results as compared to Nissen's fundoplication which is associated with higher incidence of post-surgery dysphagia.

HOW WOULD YOU INVESTIGATE IRON-DEFICIENT ANAEMIA (IDA)?

Proven iron-deficient anaemia should be investigated according to the British Society of Gastroenterology (BSG) guidelines:

➤ Confirm IDA pattern (decreased ferritin, MCV, MCH).
➤ Check coeliac serology; if positive then the patient should have an upper GI endoscopy and D2 biopsy.
➤ All patients should have OGD and colonoscopy. (Failure to reach the caecum on colonscopy should be followed up by completion barium enema.)
➤ If these are all normal, then a trial of oral iron supplementation is appropriate and then review at 3 months.
➤ If the patient remains transfusion dependant, then the small bowel should be imaged with either a small bowel study or capsule endoscopy.

WHAT ARE THE POSSIBLE CAUSES OF IRON-DEFICIENT ANAEMIA BLOOD LOSS?

➤ Aspirin/NSAIDs.
➤ Colonic cancer.
➤ Gastric cancer.
➤ Peptic ulcer disease.
➤ Small bowel tumours.
➤ Ampullary cancer.
➤ Carcinoids/Meckel's.
➤ Menstruation.
➤ Blood donation.
➤ Haematuria.
➤ Epistaxis.
➤ Coeliac disease.

Breast and endocrine

> ➤ Gynaecomastia
> ➤ Li-fraumeni syndrome
> ➤ Transplant rejection
> ➤ Drugs

GYNAECOMASTIA

How would you manage 22-year-old male who presents to clinic with suspected gynaecomastia?

➤ Take a history and perform full clinical examination.
➤ I would specifically ask about pubertal change, drug history and cannabis usage. Abdominal and testicular examination is essential.
➤ I would check FBC, LFTs and prolactin levels.

A case of gynaecomastia should be managed similar to any other breast lump and have the full triple assessment. I would arrange ultrasound, mammogram and FNAC. Core biopsy is not essential here in a young patient but is an option.

The critical points here are that you must exclude a testicular neoplasm and get a tissue sample. In a young male patient this condition usually resolves after 12–18 months and is usually physiological. If after stopping any offending drugs, options are: a trial course of tamoxifen, liposuction or a subcutaneous mastectomy.

LI-FRAUMENI SYNDROME

What is Li-Fraumeni syndrome?

Li-Fraumeni syndrome is a cancer predisposition syndrome associated with soft-tissue sarcoma, breast cancer, leukaemia, osteosarcoma, melanoma, adrenal cortex and brain. More than 50% of individuals diagnosed clinically have an identifiable diease-causing mutation in the TP53 gene. It is inherited in an autosomal dominant manner.

It is defined by the following criteria:

➤ A relative with a sarcoma diagnosed before the age of 45 AND
➤ A first-degree relative with any cancer under the age of 45 AND
➤ A first- or second-degree relative with any cancer under the age of 45 or a sarcoma at any age (Li and Fraumeni 1969).

TRANSPLANT REJECTION

Types of rejection

➤ Hyperacute rejection: a complement-mediated reaction and occurs within minutes of the transplant.
➤ Acute rejection: usually begins within 8–10 days and is highest in the first 3 months. It is caused by HLA incompatibility.
➤ Chronic rejection: occurs after 1 year.

For the general surgeon, questions around treatment of acute rejection and drug toxicities are important. Acute rejection typically occurs around 8–10 days post-op and will present with tenderness, raised WCC, rigors and raised creatinine.

Key principles of management

➤ Direct referral to specialist unit.
➤ Treat first episode of rejection with IV methylprednisolone 250 mg.

DRUGS

Taken from the Edinburgh Renal Transplant Unit Handbook (Turner *et al.*).

Tacrolimus

Administration

➤ Oral route in most instances (well absorbed even in those with NG tubes).
➤ It is administered usually at 10 a.m. and 10 p.m.
➤ The capsules are taken on an empty stomach either 1 hour before or 2–3 hours after meals.
➤ Contents of the capsule can be suspended in water for NG administration.
➤ One-fifth of the oral dose can be given as a continuous IV infusion in saline via non-PVC bags/tubing if absolutely necessary.

Levels

Whole blood trough levels to be checked on Mondays, Wednesdays and Fridays. The target level for the first 6 months is 10 ng/mL (range: 8–12 ng/mL) and 5–10 ng/mL after 6 months. In adult kidney transplant patients, steady state may be reached 2–3 days after starting therapy or changing dose.

Contraindications

Live vaccines are not to be given to immunosuppressed patients.

Tacrolimus is contraindicated in pregnancy. Since it is not known to what extent tacrolimus may influence the efficacy of oral contraceptives it is generally recommended that other forms of contraception be used.

Side-effects

The most frequent side-effects seen with tacrolimus include:
➤ abnormal kidney function (similar to ciclosporin)
➤ tremor
➤ headache
➤ parasthesiae.

Less common side-effects:
➤ diarrhoea
➤ hypertension
➤ hyperglycaemia
➤ hyperkalaemia
➤ hypomagnesaemia
➤ visual and neurological disturbances (affected patients should not drive or operate machinery)
➤ hypertrophic cardiomyopathy (in paediatric patients with trough levels >25 mg/mL).

Ciclosporin

Contraindications/cautions

➤ Live vaccines are not to be given to immunocompromised patients.
➤ Neoral should be used with caution during pregnancy.
➤ Ciclosporin passes into breast milk, so mothers should not breast-feed their infants.

Side-effects

The most frequent side-effects seen with ciclosporin include:
➤ abnormal kidney function
➤ hypertrichosis
➤ tremor
➤ hypertension
➤ hepatic dysfunction
➤ gingival hypertrophy
➤ gastrointestinal disturbances
➤ burning sensations of hands and feet.

Less common side-effects:
➤ headaches
➤ weight increase

➤ mild anaemia
➤ hyperkalaemia
➤ hyperuricaemia
➤ hypomagnasaemia
➤ hypercholesterolaemia
➤ rashes (possible allergic origin)
➤ oedema
➤ pancreatitis
➤ neuropathy
➤ reversible dysmenhorrhoea
➤ muscle weakness cramps or myopathy.

Azathioprine

Administration

Virtually exclusively oral, although an IV preparation is available.

Contraindications

➤ Pregnancy.
➤ Bone marrow dysfunction, i.e. patients who are known to be leucopaenic or thrombocytopaenic.
➤ Reduce dose if hepatic dysfunction is present.

Side-effects

➤ Bone marrow suppression – usually reversible following cessation.
➤ Cholestatis and disturbed liver function – again usually reversible.
➤ Pancreatitis.
➤ Dose may require to be altered depending on WCC, i.e. reduce if WCC <4.0, stop if WCC <3.0 and re-introduce at a lower dose when WCC >3.0.

Mycophenolate mofetil (MMF)

Current indication

As a substitute for azathioprine in alternative triple therapy regimen for patients at high risk of rejection and following resistant rejection in patients treated with standard triple therapy.

Mode of action

➤ MMF is rapidly hydrolysed following absorption to mycophenolic acid (MPA), the active metabolite.
➤ MPA is a potent inhibitor of inosine monophosphate dehydrogenase (IMPDH) and therefore inhibits the denovo pathway of guanosine nucleotide synthesis.
➤ B and T lymphocytes are critically dependant on the de novo pathway and so MPA inhibits B and T lymphocyte proliferation and also B-cell antibody formation.

Contraindications

Pregnancy.

Side-effects

➤ Neutropenia.
➤ Gastrointestinal bloating.
➤ Cramps.
➤ Diarrhoea.
➤ Vomiting.

Prednisolone

Prescription and reduction

Prednisolone is normally reduced according to the following schedule (this schedule may be altered if rejection occurs):
➤ 20 mg daily × 1 month started on day 2
➤ 15 mg daily × 1 month
➤ 10 mg daily × 1 month
➤ 5 mg daily thereafter.

All patients to receive ranitidine (150 mg od) along with prednisolone. After 3 months continue minimum of 5 mg or 7.5 mg if >75 kg in weight. Keep on maintenance dose until the end of the first year and then review.

At 1 year, cessation of prednisolone should be considered – see steroid withdrawal protocol. Caution should be exercised in patients with an 'increased risk' of rejection. Cautions relating to steroid withdrawal include:
➤ FACs +ve
➤ >2 transplants
➤ panel reactive antibodies >50%/highly sensitised patients
➤ rejection episodes >1 or more acute rejection episodes Banff grade > II
➤ late acute rejection, i.e. occurring after 6 months.

Steroid withdrawal

Steroid withdrawal should be discussed with the patient and they should be informed of the risk of rejection. The steroids should be withdrawn according to the following schedule.
➤ Decrease by 1 mg per month til 0 mg.
➤ Monthly measurements till at least 3 months after cessation.

Steroid-induced osteoporosis

All patients should receive additional elemental calcium. This may be as one or two tablets per day depending on dietary intake.
➤ If GFR >50 mLs/min Adcal-D3 (or similiar) should be used.
➤ If GFR <50 mLs/min Alfacalcidol and Calchew should be used.

Bisphosphonates

IV pamidronate may be used in the initial post-transplant period in patients with: known osteopenia or osteoporosis, a history of one or more previous transplants, two or more episodes of rejection (treated with high dose steroid therapy) or a history of previous disease management with steroids.

All patients should be given advice on

➤ Diet.
➤ Weight.
➤ Exercise.
➤ Smoking cessation.

General surgery of childhood

> ➤ Foreign body ingestion
> ➤ Bile stained vomiting
> ➤ Pyloric stenosis
> ➤ Intussusception
> ➤ Umbilical and epigastric hernia
> ➤ Inguinal hernia and hydrocoele
> ➤ The acute scrotum

FOREIGN BODY INGESTION

The exam question will be that you are the consultant general surgeon and a child, e.g. a 2-year-old, has swallowed an object. Typically it will be a 5p coin or button battery. How will you manage the case? Transferring to a paediatric centre as your answer will not be entertained. YOU must manage the case.

Key points

➤ 50% of such patients are asymptomatic.
➤ If the object has got passed cricopharyngeus, then it is likely that it will pass completely.
➤ CXR is negative in 20% cases.
➤ If the object is in the stomach and the child is well, you may safely discharge the patient.
➤ 90% of foreign bodies are coins.
➤ The children are usually 18–48 months old.
➤ Do a CXR first (this should cover neck, chest and abdomen).

The problem occurs if the object is lodged in the oesophagus.
➤ Coins lodged in the UPPER two-thirds of the oesophagus will require to be removed either endoscopically or surgically.

➤ Coins in the LOWER one-third can have a trial of conservative for 24 hours with a repeat CXR. This will have a 90% success rate.

NB: Button batteries need to be removed urgently because of the pressure necrosis effects.

The options for removal are:
➤ Foley catheter
➤ forceps
➤ basket
➤ embolectomy catheter.

Clearly, if you do not have anaesthetic facilities for this age group or you are not prepared to operate, then the child should be transferred to a paediatric surgical unit, but food bolus obstruction and foreign bodies are well within the realm of the general surgeon and are fair game for this exam.

BILE STAINED VOMITING

A scenario of bile stained vomiting in the general FRCS exam will only be there to test your recognition of its importance. This is clearly the domain of the specialist paediatric surgeon and you will not be expected to be able to manage this patient.

You will be expected to recognise the importance and manage the initial investigations and resuscitation.

Key points
➤ Bile stained vomiting is a surgical emergency.
➤ The baby has malrotation volvulus till proven otherwise.
➤ Fluid resuscitation should begin immediately.
➤ A plain AXR is the first investigation followed by contrast swallow.
➤ NG tube.
➤ Transfer to specialist paediatric centre.

PYLORIC STENOSIS

Effortless, non-bilious vomiting in an infant 3–5 weeks of age is the typical presentation of infantile hypertrophic pyloric stenosis (IHPS).

Typical features
➤ Infant aged 3–8 weeks (very uncommon <3 weeks).
➤ Firstborn male child, four times more common in males.
➤ Non-bilious projectile vomiting.
➤ Hypochloraemic, hypokalaemic metabolic alkalosis.
➤ Family history: increased risk in first-degree relative, especially if incident case is female.

Diagnosis

The typical palpable mass is firm, mobile, 1–2 cm and best palpated from the left, located in the mid-epigastrum beneath the liver edge.
➤ Diagnosis by palpation alone only successful in 50% cases.
➤ Ultrasound features:
  ➢ pyloric wall thickness >4 mm
  ➢ pyloric canal length >14 mm.
➤ Differential diagnosis: overfeeding (>120–150 mL/kg/day), GORD, viral gastroenteritis.

Treatment

➤ Slow correction of metabolic abnormalities.
➤ Can normally be achieved without fluid bolus.
➤ 150 mL/kg/24 hours 0.45% NaCl, 5% dextrose, 10–20 mmol KCL is standard fluid resuscitation regime.
➤ Aim for bicarbonate <30 mmol/L.
➤ Normalise chloride.
➤ NG tube may be used but may drive gastric losses (should always be in situ for transfer).
➤ Ramstedt's pyloromyotomy.
➤ Laparoscopic pyloromyotomy.

The first priority in treating an infant with pyloric stenosis is to correct the fluid and electrolyte inbalance. This is achieved with 0.45% saline with potassium over 1–2 days. There is no role for emergency surgery and antibiotics are not normally required. The traditional approach to the pylorus is through a right upper quadrant incision. Newer approaches are by laparoscopy or a peri-umbilical approach. The postoperative course is usually uneventful and most patients can be discharged within 2–3 days. Opinions vary regarding when to start feeding but it is usually not within 4 hours of surgery. There is no evidence that half-strength feeds/delayed feeding decreases length of hospital stay.

Vomiting may persist post surgery due to oedema within the pylorus; this is expected to settle by day 4–5. If vomiting is troublesome or persistant, then an incomplete myotomy must be considered and ruled out by contrast exam. A further myotomy or balloon dilation is considered primarily on clinical grounds. A healthy feeding baby on discharge may not require follow-up.

INTUSSUSCEPTION

Definition: This is the invagination of the intestine into itself in a distal direction.
➤ It is usually caused by hypertrophied peyers patch. It has a 1% mortality and occurs in about 1 in 1000 live births. It most commonly occurs between 3 months and 1 year with a peak presentation at 6 months.
➤ Typically there is a history of upper respiratory chest infection or

gastroenteritis and presents with sudden onset of severe colicky abdominal pain and vomiting. Classical features are drawing the legs up into the abdomen and the passage of redcurrant jelly stool. These episodes last up to 20 minutes.
➤ The diagnosis is made by ultrasound.
➤ The initial management is:
  ➢ IV fluid resuscitation
  ➢ antibiotics
  ➢ NG tube
  ➢ pneumatic reduction is 80% successful.
➤ A surgeon should be present for pneumatic reduction in case of perforation as this will cause rapid and severe abdominal distension, similar to a tension pneumothorax and will require immediate decompression.

A laparotomy will be required for:
➤ septicaemia
➤ perforation
➤ peritonitis
➤ failed reduction.

UMBILICAL AND EPIGASTRIC HERNIA
Umbilical hernias are common presentations to surgical outpatients. A true umbilical hernia in a child will usually close spontaneously by the age of 2 years. Any umbilical hernia presenting up to this age should be reassured and managed conservatively. If the hernia persists after this then surgical repair is warranted. An open procedure should be performed and done without a mesh.

Epigastric hernia on the otherhand should be fixed. These have a higher rate of obstruction and should be placed on the elective waiting list.

INGUINAL HERNIA AND HYDROCOELE
What is a hydrocoele?
➤ A hydrocoele is a collection of fluid around the testicle (testis), in the tunica vaginalis (the space surrounding the testis).
➤ Hydrocoeles only occur in males.
➤ Typically presents as a painless swelling of the scrotum.
➤ Most hydrocoeles are congenital (i.e. present at birth) – these are usually seen in boys aged 1–2 years of age. Most congenital hydrocoeles resolve by the end of the first year of life. Persistent congenital hydrocoele is readily corrected surgically.
➤ Secondary hydrocoeles can affect males of any age, but usually occur in men older than 40 years.
➤ May affect one side of the scrotum or both sides.

Causes of hydrocoeles in adults

In many cases, no cause is found. Possible causes include:

➤ trauma – traumatic hydrocoeles are common
➤ infection (e.g. epididymo-orchitis)
➤ testicular tumour
➤ torsion of the testes – reactive hydocoeles occur in up to 20% of cases of testicular torsion.

Symptoms of a hydrocoele

➤ Painless, enlarged scrotum.
➤ There may be a sensation of heaviness or dragging.
➤ Hydrocoele is not usually painful (pain may be an indication of an accompanying infection).

Investigations

➤ A light shined through the scrotum will cause the hydrocoele to illuminate (transillumination).
➤ Investigation is not usually required in children.
➤ For adults, an ultrasound of the testis may be required.

Since testicular lumps could potentially be missed on physical examination (due to the collection of fluid preventing full examination of the testis), an ultrasound is often advised. An ultrasound of the scrotum will confirm the diagnosis of hydrocoele and also identify any abnormal testicular lumps.

Treatment of hydrocoeles:

➤ If the hydrocoele is small, no treatment is usually required.
➤ For larger hydrocoeles, drawing off of the fluid using a needle and syringe may be indicated. However, such needle aspiration is not therapeutic because the fluid generally reaccumulates quickly and is associated with a risk of infection.
➤ For larger hydrocoeles, or where there is a suspected underlying tumour, surgery may be required.
➤ Hydrocoeles can usually be cured with a relatively simple surgical operation.

NB: Most hydrocoeles occur with normal testes. However, always see your doctor if you notice any change in the size and/or shape of your scrotum or testes.

TESTICULAR TORSION

This occurs in 1 in 4000 males and accounts for 30% of cases of the acute scrotum. The typical age is peri-pubertal. It typically presents with the sudden onset of groin pain and vomiting. Clinically, there may be a tender, swollen red testicle. The cremasteric reflex is normally absent. Urgent surgical exploration is required within 4–6 hours.

The differential diagnosis includes:

➤ Testicular torsion: 30% of cases, 10–25 years old.
➤ Hydatid of Morgagni: 50% of cases, 6–12 years old.
➤ Idiopathic scrotal oedema: 5% of cases, 2–10 years old.
➤ Epidydimitis: 5% cases.

The exam question here is that a 12-year-old boy is admitted with acute onset of right-sided testicular pain. How will you manage the case?

The key points are that testicular torsion must be excluded and urgent scrotal exploration must be performed. The examiners may try to push you into getting an ultrasound or delaying his surgery till the next NCEPOD list. The answer is that if you suspect a torsion, you operate immediately. A testicular torsion should be treated with the same urgency as a ruptured aortic aneurysm.

➤ Bleeding from an incision in the tunica albuginea is the best prognostic sign for viability.
➤ Necrotic tissue = orchidectomy.
➤ Contra-lateral orchidopexy with 4/0 Prolene.
➤ Delay any prosthesis insertion for 6/12 or puberty.

Critical care and emergency surgery

> ➤ Oxygen delivery and monitoring
> ➤ Sepsis
> ➤ Inotropes
> ➤ Blood transfusion
> ➤ Renal failure
> ➤ Anaesthetic procedures
> ➤ Hypothermia
> ➤ Brain stem death
> ➤ Nutrition/TPN
> ➤ Abdominal compartment syndrome
> ➤ Postoperative care
> ➤ Key emergency cases
> ➤ Diathermy
> ➤ Miscellaneous Viva questions

OXYGEN DELIVERY AND MONITORING
How does a pulse oximeter work?

Pulse oximetry is a simple non-invasive method of monitoring the percentage of haemoglobin (Hb) that is saturated with oxygen. A source of light originates from the probe at two wavelengths (650 nm and 805 nm). The light is partly absorbed by haemoglobin, by amounts that differ depending on whether it is saturated or desaturated with oxygen. By calculating the absorption at the two wavelengths the processor can compute the proportion of haemoglobin that is oxygenated. The oximeter is dependant on a pulsatile flow and produces a graph of the quality of the flow.

The pulse oximeter is accurate in the range of oxygen saturations 70–100%, but less accurate under 70%.

In the following situations the pulse oximeter readings may not be accurate:

➤ A reduction in peripheral pulsatile blood flow produced by peripheral vasoconstriction (hypovolaemia, severe hypotension, cold, cardiac failure, some cardiac arrhythmias) or peripheral vascular disease.
➤ Venous congestion, particularly when caused by tricuspid regurgitation.
➤ Bright overhead lights in theatre.
➤ Shivering.
➤ Pulse oximetry cannot distinguish between different forms of haemoglobin. Carbo-oxyhaemoglobin (haemoglobin combined with carbon monoxide) is registered as 90% oxygenated haemoglobin and 10% desaturated haemoglobin and therefore the oximeter will overestimate the saturation.
➤ Nail varnish may cause falsely low reading.

NB: These units are NOT affected by jaundice, dark skin or anaemia.
   Oximeters give no information about the level of CO_2, and therefore have limitations in the assessment of patients developing respiratory failure due to CO_2 retention. (Refer to: www.nda.ox.ac.uk)

SEPSIS
What is meant by the term SIRS?
Systemic inflammatory response syndrome (SIRS) is a non-specific manifestation and may be diagnosed if at least two of the following criteria are met:
➤ temp >38°C or <36°C
➤ tachycardia >90 bpm
➤ tachypnoea >20 resp/min
➤ white cell count >12 or <4.

SIRS differs from sepsis in that sepsis is SIRS with a documented infection.
   Septic shock is sepsis with refractory arterial hypotension and/or need for inotropes despite adequate fluid resuscitation.
   The physiological changes occurring in patients with severe sepsis and septic shock are myriad and include changes that are clearly detrimental such as decreased contractility of the left and right ventricle, increased venous capacitance, increased pulmonary vascular resistance, and capillary leak. Increased ventricular compliance and sinus tachycardia are likely adaptive responses allowing the ventricle to maintain, and even manifest increased cardiac input, following volume resuscitation despite decreased contractility. The decreased arteriolar resistance may also be adaptive, although when profound, produces detrimental and potentially lethal hypotension.

What do you understand by the term 'early goal-directed therapy' (EGDT)?

The recommendations for initial resuscitation are centred around the Rivers trial (2001) of early goal-directed therapy, which showed significant improvement in (a) hospital mortality, (b) 28-day mortality and (c) 60-day mortality.

How do you manage septicaemia and septic shock?

These patients are often pale, acidotic, hypotensive, cyanosed and confused. The mortality is considerable and if the patient develops septic shock, may be in excess of 50%. This is as true of Gram-positive as Gram-negative bacteraemia, as the cytokine cascade leads to DIC with multi-organ disease and septic shock arises with both varieties of infection.

The patients are usually febrile and hypotensive, with a BP of <90 systolic – but may be apyrexial but tachycardia. The white cell count may be raised – but many patients are often neutropenic and this is often a poor prognostic indicator. The platelet count may be low, and if so, the patient may have DIC. The commonest sources of infection are chest, gut, biliary tree, soft tissue and urine.

After FBC, biochemistry, INR and clotting, glucose, and CXR have been performed, blood cultures (at least two sets) should be taken. Look carefully for obvious sources of infection, i.e: urine/throat/CSF/abscess/high vaginal swab/sputum/stool/joint/leg ulcer.

An IV infusion should be set up immediately with crystalloid. If the BP remains low, below 100 mmHg systolic in spite of this initial management plus 'best guess' antimicrobial chemotherapy and oxygen, then this patient should be considered for treatment with inotropes and tranfered to a high dependence unit pending furthur investigation.

How would you manage a 75-year-old diabetic man who presents to the vascular ward with wet gangrene, BP 80 and poor urine output?

➤ ABC.
➤ Oxygen.
➤ IV access.
➤ Bloods/blood cultures.
➤ ABG.
➤ CXR and X-ray foot.
➤ IV antibiotics.
➤ Insulin sliding scale.
➤ Admit patient to HDU.
➤ Inotropic support (see questions on choice of inotrope).
➤ Central and arterial line.
➤ Theatre (see question on how to do BKA).

What are the clinically important organisms in surgery?
Gram +ve Cocci

Staphylococci
➤ *Staphylococcus aureus* (coagulase positive).
➤ *Staphylococcus epidermidis* (coagulase positive).

Streptococci
These may be classified as alpha-, beta- or non-haemolytic by the Lancefield classification.
➤ Beta-haemolytic streptococci:
  ➢ *Streptococcus pyogenes* (Group A).
➤ Alpha-haemolytic streptococci:
  ➢ *Streptococcus mitior*
  ➢ *Streptococcus pneumonia*
  ➢ *Streptococcus sanguis.*
➤ Non-haemolytic streptococci:
  ➢ *Streptococcus bovis*
  ➢ *Enterococcus.*

Gram-positive bacilli (rods)
➤ Aerobic:
  ➢ *Bacillus anthracis*
  ➢ *Listeria monocytogenes.*
➤ Anaerobic:
  ➢ *Clostridium botulinum*
  ➢ *Clostridium perfringes*
  ➢ *Clostridium tetani*
  ➢ *Clostridium difficile.*

Infection of skin and soft tissue
Staphylococcus aureus is the principle organism causing suppuration, and recurrent abscesses can occur even if antibiotics are used.

Cellulitis may present with generalised erythema, increased oedema, bullae and lymphangitis. There may be systemic signs of fevers, rigors and confusion suggesting bacteraemia. Common causative organisms are *Streptococcus pyogenes*, *Staphylococcus aureus* and *Pseudomonas aeruginosa*.

Necrotising fasciitis
This is a rare and life-threatening condition. The lower limbs and groin are the most commonly affected, with patients exhibiting pain, swelling and fever on admission. Tenderness, erythema and warm skin are the early signs. Small bullae develop as the infection progresses and bullae with serous fluid are characteristic. Late signs are large haemorrhagic bullae, necrosis, fluctuance and crepitus. There may be minimal signs of cutaneous infection initially, but

extensive destruction of the subcutaneous tissues with bacteraemia, septic shock, multiple organ failure and death may soon follow.

Risk and predisposing factors are:

➤ diabetes (the most common)
➤ alcoholism
➤ IVDAs
➤ immunosuppression
➤ HIV
➤ steroids
➤ malnutrition
➤ liver disease
➤ renal failure
➤ obesity.

Fournier's gangrene is a form of necrotising fasciitis involving the scrotum and perineum. When it involves the abdominal wall it is called Meleney's gangrene.

Gram-negative cocci

➤ *Neisseria meningitides.*
➤ *Neisseria gonorrhea.*

Gram-positive bacilli

➤ *Escherichia coli.*
➤ *Proteus mirabilis.*
➤ *Klebsiella.*
➤ *Salmonella.*
➤ *Shigella.*
➤ *Haemophilus influenza.*
➤ *Pseudomonas aeruginosa.*
➤ *Vibrio cholera.*
➤ *Campylobacter jejuni.*
➤ *Helicobacter pylori.*

Which antibiotic?

Metronidazole 500 mg tds iv
Good anaerobic cover. Used almost universally for prophylaxis in bowel surgery. Also given orally to treat *C. difficile* (poor gastrointestinal absorption).

Cephalosporins, normally ceftriaxone 1g iv od
Broad-spectrum gram-negative antimicrobial properties. Recent controversy around *C. difficile* infections. Use with caution in high-risk groups (elderly/ nursing home residents).

Gentamycin 7 mg/kg daily (aminoglycoside)

Broad-spectrum bactericidal antimicrobial but inactive against anaerobes and has poor activity against haemolytic streptococci and pneumococci. Best used for staph or Gram-negative infections. Given blind for serious infections, e.g. acute diverticulitis is usually given with a B-lactam +/– metronnidazole. Narrow therapeutic window; nephrotoxic at high doses. Requires freqent level monitoring. Can precipitate renal failure.

Ciprofloxacin 500 mg bd

Active against Gram-positive and Gram-negative organisms. Particularly active against Gram-negative bacteria including *Salmonella*, *Shigella*, *Campylobacter*, *Neisseria* and *Pseudomonas*. Oral dose gives similar bioavailability to IV.

Flucloxacillin 500 mg qds

Active against *S. Aureus*. Used in treatment on simple abscesses/cellulitis. Good oral bioavailability.

Benzylpenicillin 500 mg qds (can be increased in severe infection)

Active against *Streptococci species*. Used for skin/soft tissue infection but also in disseminated infection, i.e. septic arthritris/endocaridits. Not active orally, phenoxymethylpenicillin is the oral alternative.

Augmentin 1.2g tds iv

Amoxicillin with clavulanic acid. Active against anaerobes and penicillinase-producing organisms. Common cause of cholestatic jaundice and frequently causes diarrhoea. Also associated with *C. difficile* infection.

Second line agents
Vancomycin 125 mg qds po/1g daily iv

First line agent against *C. difficile,* given orally. Intravenous dose for severe staphylococcal infections in those who are penicillin allergic. Prophylaxis in graft prosthesis in vascular surgery.

Tazocin 4.5g tds iv

Active against enterococci. First line agent for cholecystitis and diverticulitis. Secreted in bile.

Neutropenic sepsis

Risk depends upon:
- degree of neutropenia:
  - <0.5 = significant risk
  - <0.2 = very high risk.
- duration of neutropenia >7 days is a significant risk.

May present with rigors, chest infection, pneumonia, cellulitis, UTI, septic shock.

Do FBC, U+E, LFTs, CXR, microbiology swabs, blood cultures, clotting.

Rx:
> ABC/resuscitation
> broad-spectrum antibiotics, e.g. tazocin and gentamycin
> if no response in 48 hours, add Gram-positive cover, e.g. vancomycin/ teicoplainin
> if no response at 72 hours, add IV antifungal, e.g. caspofungin.

Discuss postoperative infections

Surgical site infection

Bacteria are usually associated with surgical site infection, but *Candida* may be isolated. *Staphlococcus aureus* is the most common isolate, even after colonic surgery, although enterococcus and coagulase-negative staphylococci are also commonly isolated.

Surgical site infection can also be caused by enteric bacteria, e.g. *E. coli*, *Proteus mirabilis*, *Klebsiella*, in synergy with anaerobes, particularly after colonic surgery. Gram-negative bacteria can infect surgical site infections opportunistically.

What are the NICE Guidelines on Surgical Site Infection (SSI)?

Surgical site infections (SSI) comprise 20% of all healthcare-associated infections. At least 5% of patients undergoing surgery develop a surgical site infection. NICE guidelines Surgical Site Infection 2008 state:

Preoperative phase
> Advise patients to have shower or bath prior to surgery.
> If hair has to be removed, use electric clippers with a single-use disposable head on the day of surgery.
> Do not use razors for hair removal, because they increase the risk of SSI.
> Do not give antibiotic prophylaxis routinely for clean surgery.
> Give a repeat dose (if used), if the operation is longer than the half-life of the antibiotic.
> Staff preparation.

Intraoperative phase
> Wear sterile gowns.
> Nail brush prior to first operation of the list.
> Prep skin with either povidone-iodine or chlorhexidine.
> Maintain patient homeostasis (temperature, optimal oxygenation, adequate perfusion).
> Dressings.
> Do not use incise drapes except IOBAN.

➤ Do not use diathermy for skin incision.
➤ Do not use wound irrigation.

Postoperative phase
➤ Do not use topical antimicrobial agents for surgical wounds.
➤ Do not use moist cotton gauze for surgical wounds that are healing by secondary intention.

Hospital-acquired infections?
In the current climate of political correctness, you can expect some sort of question based on this. The usual suspects are *C. diff* and MRSA.

Clostridium difficile is a Gram-positive anaerobic bacteria. It is a normal commensal in approximately 2–5% of the population. In children, however, it can be present in up to 70% of normal gut flora. It produces in susceptible patients two toxins: enterotoxin (toxin A) and cytotoxin (toxin B). It is transmitted from person to person via the faecal–oral route. It can be cultured from almost any surface in the hospital.

Risk factors
➤ Antibiotics.
➤ Renal failure.
➤ ICU.
➤ Elderly.
➤ Prolonged stay in hospital.
➤ Comorbidity.

Treatment
➤ Oral vancomycin 125 mg QDS.
➤ Oral/IV metronidazole.

The typical exam question here will be along the lines of: 'You are asked to see an elderly patient on a medical ward with diarrhoea'.
The following lines of questions will then follow:
➤ What are the causes of diarrhoea?
➤ How will you assess the patient?
➤ What tests would you order?
➤ What would be your clinical concerns?

This discussion will then rapidly follow on to a scenario of *C. diff* colitis and how you will proceed. You will be asked:
➤ How will you assess the patient?
➤ What investigations will you use?
➤ When will you operate?

All these questions are focused around the use of rigid sigmoidoscopy and biopsy of a pseudomembrane, diameter of colon in toxicity and what operation you will do at laparotomy.

Key principles revolve around perioperative management and the decision YOU are going to make about when and how to take the colon out.
➤ Daily bloods and clinical examination.
➤ Daily AXR (>6 cm diameter = toxic megacolon).
➤ Ideally, should be joint care with GI physicians.
➤ IV steroids and fluid resuscitation.

Indications for surgery
➤ Generalised peritonitis.
➤ Free air under the diaphragm.
➤ Toxic colon on AXR.
➤ Failed medical treatment.

The operation to be done is a subtotal colectomy and end ileostomy.

INOTROPES
Tell me about inotropes
Classification of inotropes
cAMP dependant:
➤ beta-adrenergic receptor agonists
➤ phosphodiesterase inhibitors
➤ glucagon.

cAMP independent:
➤ alpha-receptor agonists
➤ dopexamine
➤ cardiac gylcosides
➤ thyroid hormone
➤ calcium.

Adrenergic receptors
➤ Alpha-1 adrenergic receptor:
  ➢ arteriolar vasoconstriction
  ➢ increased inotropic effect.
➤ Alpha-2 adrenergic receptor:
  ➢ peripheral vasoconstrition.
➤ Beta-1 adrenergic receptor:
  ➢ increased inotropic effect
  ➢ increased chronotropic effect.
➤ Beta-2 adrenergic receptor:
  ➢ bronchodilation
  ➢ (K, Ca, Mg) shift.

When do you use inotropes?

Adrenaline

➤ Alpha and beta.
➤ Beta-receptor agonism > alpha effect.
➤ 0.01 – 1.0 µg/kg/min.
➤ Major use: when you need A and B:
  ➢ resuscitation
  ➢ arrhythmias/tachycardia.
  ➢ hyperglycaemia.

Noradrenaline

➤ Alpha and beta.
➤ Predominant alpha agonist.
➤ 0.02–3.0 µg/kg/min.
➤ Major use: when you need A and B.
➤ Drug of choice for septic shock.
➤ Increases SVR (peripheral vasoconstriction).

Dopamine

➤ Dopaminergic, beta, alpha.
➤ Biochemical precursor to noradrenaline and adrenaline.
➤ Dopa: 1–5 mg/kg/min.
➤ Possibly increases renal blood flow.
➤ Beta: 5–10 µg/kg/min.
➤ Inotropy/chronotropy.
➤ Alpha: >10 µg/kg/min.
➤ Vasoconstriction.

Dobutamine

➤ Racemic mixture of (+) and (−) isomers.
➤ Mainly beta-1 receptor agonist.
➤ Inotropic/chronotropic.
➤ 2–20 µg/kg/min.
➤ Major use: systolic dysfunction.
➤ Cardiac parameters increased.

BLOOD TRANSFUSION

What are the complications of a massive blood transfusion?

A massive blood transfusion is defined as the entire blood volume replaced
within a 24-hour period. The complications are:
➤ dilutional coagulopathy
➤ hypothermia
➤ reduced 2,3-DPG due to storage, shifting dissociation curve to the LEFT
➤ hypocalcaemia (due to citrate toxicity)

➤ hyperkalaemia
➤ haemolysis
➤ transfusion-related acute lung injury (TRALI)
➤ transfusion reactions
➤ infections (virus, malaria, prions)
➤ metabolic acidosis.

When do you transfuse blood?

The decision to transfuse any patient for a given indication must balance the risks of not transfusing. In a haemodynamically stable patient, one unit of concentrated red cells should be transfused at a time, allowing the benefit of each to be assessed at 24-hourly intervals.

Where possible, anaemia should be corrected prior to major surgery, to reduce the exposure to allogenic transfusion. During the intraoperative period the use of blood must reflect the ongoing rate of surgical blood loss, continued haemodynamic instability, and anticipated postoperative bleeding.

Regarding postoperative thresholds, one can follow the SIGN guidelines, which state that transfusion is required at haemoglobin levels <70 g/dL. Patients with cardiovascular disease, or those expected to have a high incidence of covert cardiovascular disease such as the elderly are likely to benefit from transfusion when their haemoglobin levels fall below 90 g/dL. Transfusion is not indicated at values >100 g/dL.

What are the clinical features of acute transfusion reactions?

➤ Pyrexia.
➤ GI (nausea, vomiting, diarrhoea).
➤ Respiratory (dyspnoea, wheeze, cough, cyanosis).
➤ Cardiac (hypotension, tachycardia).
➤ Renal (oliguria).
➤ CNS (anxiety, confusion, restlessness).
➤ Systemic (myalgia, chest pain, pruritus, arthralgia).

The possibility of an acute transfusion reaction should be suspected if any of these features develop for the first time during or shortly after a transfusion.

What are the immediate steps in the management of a suspected acute transfusion reaction?

➤ Stop the transfusion.
➤ ABC.
➤ In full anaphylactic shock, dial 2222 and give adrenaline.
➤ Check vital signs.
➤ Check sample ID.
➤ Exclude ABO incompatibility.
➤ Take repeat bloods and blood cultures.
➤ Discuss case with BTS.

In the case of full anaphylactic shock, the initial diagnosis is usually reached on clinical grounds. In the majority of other cases the clinical features combined with subsequent investigations will help to identify the cause.

In febrile non-haemolytic transfusion reaction (FNHTR), the patient usually has a history of previous transfusion and/or multiple pregnancies. It usually occurs within 30 minutes or longer after starting, but can occur 1–2 hours after the transfusion has been completed. Typically the patient is generally not unwell. Rigors and/or chills may occur in abscence of pyrexia. Always distinguish from the early stages of ABO incompatibility and septicaemia due to underlying disease or to transfusion.

In acute haemolytic transfusion reaction, it is almost invariably with a red cell transfusion. The most common cause of this reaction is a clerical error and patient misidentification, i.e. the patient receiving the wrong blood. This reaction is usually rapid after 100 mL of blood. The patient may have signs of shock, DIC and renal failure. This may be clinically indistinguishable from sepsis.

In transfusion-associated septicaemia, again this is clinically indistinguishable from ABO incompatibility and presents with pyrexia and shock.

Transfusion-related acute lung injury (TRALI) is relatively more common with, but not restricted to FFP and platelet transfusion. It may occur 1–6 hours after starting a transfusion but frequently starts 1–2 hours after. Typically presents with severe dyspnoea and hypoxia and features of pulmonary oedema both clinically and on CXR. There is no peripheral oedema or raised JVP. CXR features may initially be patchy and asymmetrical but no cardiomegaly or upper zone venous diversion.

RENAL FAILURE
How do you manage renal failure?
Causes:
➤ Pre-renal: 40–70%
➤ Renal: 10–50%
➤ Post-renal (obstruction): 10%.

Management
➤ No specific treatment of ARF (mainly supportive):
  ➢ dopamine
  ➢ insulin-like growth factor
  ➢ natriuretic peptides.
➤ Treat shock (but don't fluid overload).
➤ Treat sepsis.
➤ Exclude obstruction – catheter, USS.
➤ Stop nephrotoxic drugs, NSAIDs, aminoglycosides, ACE inhibitor, etc.
➤ Regular monitoring of fluid balance/weight.
➤ Consider dialysis for uraemic patients.

Complications

➤ Hyperkalaemia:
  ➤ IV insulin and glucose
  ➤ IV calcium
  ➤ metabolic acidosis/types/anion gap
  ➤ pulmonary oedema
  ➤ oxygen
  ➤ furosemide.

Management of serum potassium 6.5

➤ ABC.
➤ IV calcium (10 mL of 10% over 10 minutes) – rule of 10s.
➤ Insulin and dextrose (15 units actrapid).
➤ Salbutamol nebulisers.
➤ Calcium resonium.

ANAESTHETIC PROCEDURES

What is the ASA grade?

ASA I – Normal healthy individual.
ASA II – Mild systemic disease that does not limit activity.
ASA III – Severe systemic disease that limits activity but is not incapacitating.
ASA IV – Incapacitating systemic disease which is constantly life-threatening.
ASA V – Moribund, not expected to survive 24 hours with or without surgery.

How would you insert a central line?

Key points

➤ Indications.
➤ Anatomical landmarks.
➤ Dose of lignocaine.
➤ Complications.
➤ Central line sepsis.

What are the complications of a central line?

Having a method for classifying complications is useful and looks good in front of examiners. One way is to list the complications of the central line in the order of which the line is inserted and the structures that may be encountered as the line is inserted over the guidewire.

➤ Arterial puncture/haematoma.
➤ Air embolism.
➤ Venous thrombosis.
➤ Pneumothorax.
➤ Thoracic duct injury (left side).
➤ Sepsis.
➤ Nerve damage.

➤ Arrthymia.
➤ Endocarditis.
➤ Systemic embolism.

How would you insert a chest drain?
Key points
➤ Indications.
➤ Landmarks.
➤ Dose of local.
➤ Complications.
➤ Daily management.

Epidurals and their complications
➤ Epidural anaesthesia is a form of regional anaesthesia involving injection of drugs through a catheter placed into the epidural space. The injection can cause both a loss of sensation (anaesthesia) and a loss of pain (analgesia), by blocking the transmission of signals through nerves in or near the spinal cord.
➤ The epidural space is the space inside the bony spinal canal but outside the membrane called the dura mater (sometimes called the 'dura'). In contact with the inner surface of the dura is another membrane called the arachnoid mater ('arachnoid'). The arachnoid encompasses the cerebrospinal fluid that surrounds the spinal cord.
➤ Spinal anaesthesia is a technique whereby a local anaesthetic drug is injected into the cerebrospinal fluid.
➤ For a prolonged effect, a continuous infusion of drugs may be employed. A common solution for epidural infusion in childbirth or for postoperative analgesia is 0.2% ropivacaine or 0.125% bupivacaine, with 2 µg/mL of fentanyl added. This solution is infused at a rate between 4 and 14 mL/hour, following a loading dose to initiate the nerve block.

What is the block level?
➤ Typically, the effects of the epidural are noted below a specific level on the body (dermatome). This level (the 'block height') is chosen by the anaesthetist. The level is usually 3–4 dermatomes higher than the point of insertion. A very high insertion level may result in sparing of very low dermatomes.
➤ The intensity of the block is determined by the concentration of local anaesthetic drugs used. For example, 15 mL 0.1% bupivacaine may provide good analgesia for a woman in labour, but would likely be insufficient for surgery. Conversely, 15 mL of 0.5% bupivacaine would provide a more intense block, likely sufficient for surgery. Since the volume used in each case is the same, the spread of drug, and hence the block height, is likely to be similar.

Benefits

➤ Good analgesia with less need for systemic opiates.
➤ Reduced chest complication/infections.
➤ Reduced post-op MI.
➤ Decreased stress response to surgery.
➤ Improved gut motility.
➤ Decreased blood transfusion requirement.

Complications

➤ Block failure (5%).
➤ Bloody tap (epidural haematoma).
➤ Dural puncture and headache.
➤ High block (higher than T4).
➤ Epidural abscess.
➤ Paraplegia/arachnoiditis.

What are the contraindications for an epidural?

➤ Spina bifida.
➤ Spinal surgery.
➤ Aortic stenosis.
➤ Coagulopathy/warfarin.
➤ Sepsis/cellulitis.
➤ Raised ICP.

HYPOTHERMIA

Complications of hypothermia?

Hypothermia is defined as core body temp <35°C.

The factors that increase a patient's susceptibility to cold are:

➤ age (infancy, elderly)
➤ malnutrition
➤ endocrine (hypoglycaemia, hypothyroid, diabetes)
➤ cardiac (peripheral vascular disease)
➤ CNS (peripheral neuropathy)
➤ trauma (falls)
➤ immobility.

Infants have a high ratio of body surface area to mass, and elderly people have a decreased capacity for metabolic heat production and vasoconstriction. Less body fat decreases tissue insulation. Malnutrition and exertion decrease the fuel available for heat generation. In addition, alcohol inhibits shivering, perhaps by causing hypoglycaemia, and causes cutaneous vasodilation, which counteracts the thermoregulatory response. Endocrine conditions such as hypothyroidism, adrenal insufficiency and hypoglycaemia are accompanied by decreased metabolic heat production. People with diabetes mellitus may have peripheral or autonomic neuropathy. Autonomic neuropathy impairs reflex peripheral vasoconstriction. Central nervous system degeneration, trauma, or neoplasms may affect the hypothalamic regulatory centre.

Cold damages tissues through cellular injury and vascular impairment. Cellular injury may be due to intracellular water crystallisation, temperature-induced protein changes and membrane damage. Vasoconstriction, endothelial injury and thromboembolism contribute to vascular insuffiency and ischaemia. Vasoconstriction causes hypoperfusion and stasis.

Regarding the systemic effects, fluid sequestration in damaged tissue may cause volume depletion. Despite a decreased GFR a 'cold diuresis' may occur. Acidosis may be caused by a combination of lactic and respiratory acidosis. Shock may occur after re-warming and ischaemia may lead to rhabdomyolysis.

The systemic effects are:

➤ Mild (>32°C):
  ➢ thermoregulatory response
  ➢ hypertension
  ➢ tachycardia
  ➢ ileus
  ➢ bladder atony
  ➢ shivering
  ➢ peripheral vasoconstriction.
➤ Moderate (<32°C):
  ➢ shivering lost
  ➢ J-waves
  ➢ bradycardia
  ➢ arrhythmias
  ➢ respiratory acidosis
  ➢ V/Q mismatch
  ➢ pneumonia
  ➢ acidosis
  ➢ rhabdomyolysis
  ➢ DIC/coagulopathy.

Treatment
➤ ABC.
➤ Warm fluids.
➤ Peritoneal lavage.
➤ Bear-hugger.

BRAIN STEM DEATH
How do you confirm brain stem death?
Diagnosis of BSD

Preconditions:
➤ The patient must be comatose for >6 hours.
➤ There should be no doubt that the patient's condition is due to irremediable brain damage of known aetiology.
➤ There is no evidence that this state is due to depressant drugs.
➤ Primary hypothermia as the cause of unconsciousness must have been excluded (temperature: >35°C).
➤ Potentially reversible circulatory, metabolic and endocrine disturbances excluded.
➤ The patient is being maintained on a ventilator because spontaneous ventilation has been insufficient or has ceased altogether.

Brain stem testing: response to pain
➤ No motor responses within the cranial nerve distribution can be elicited by adequate stimulation of any somatic area. There is no limb response to supra-orbital pressure.

Brain stem testing: cranial nerves
➤ Pupillary light reflex (fixed and non-reactive).
➤ Corneal reflex (abscent bilaterally).
➤ Vestibulo-ocular reflex.
➤ Oculo-cephalic reflex (doll's eye).
➤ No gag reflex.

Brain stem testing-apnoea test
➤ No respiratory movements occur when the patient is disconnected from the mechanical ventilator.
➤ PaCO$_2$ should reach 6.7 kPa.
➤ Hypoxia prevented by pre-oxygenation.

Brain stem testing: who?
➤ Must be made by at least two medical practitioners:
  ➢ registered for at least 5 years
  ➢ are competent in this field
  ➢ are not members of the transplant team
  ➢ at least one must be a consultant.
➤ Repetition of testing and time of death.
➤ Time of death is time of FIRST test.

NUTRITION/TPN

What are the indications and complications of TPN?

Indications

➤ Ileus post major bowel surgery.
➤ Enterocutaneous fistula.
➤ Small bowel syndrome.
➤ Malabsoption syndromes.
➤ ARDS.
➤ Post oesophajectomy.
➤ Severe catabolic states.

Complications

➤ Central line sepsis.
➤ Hyperglycaemia.
➤ Altered gut flora.
➤ Bacterial translocation.
➤ Acute gastric ulceration.
➤ Liver dysfunction.

What is refeeding syndrome

Refeeding syndrome is defined as 'The occurrence of severe fluid and electrolyte shifts and their associated complications in malnourished patients undergoing refeeding either orally, enterally, or parenterally' (Solomon 1990).

It is potentially very dangerous and can lead to Wernicke's encephalopathy, cardiac arrest or death.

The high-risk categories are:

➤ chronic alcoholism
➤ chronic malnutrition
➤ anorexia nervosa
➤ marasmus
➤ patients nil by mouth for more than 7–10 days
➤ BMI <16
➤ <15% weight loss over 6 months.

The above then may lead to:

➤ hypophosphataemia
➤ hypocalcaemia
➤ hypomagnesaemia
➤ altered glucose metabolism
➤ fluid balance abnormailites.

The patient with suspected refeeding syndrome should be referred to the dietician and enteral tube feeding should be introduced at a maximum of 10 kcal/kg/day, increasing slowly to gradually meet requirements. Bloods should be done daily for 4 days until stable then twice weekly.

At-risk patients should be given thiamine as IV Pabrinex during the first 2 days of feeding. Potassium, phosphate and magnesium levels should be replaced using either oral or IV supplementation. Options are Kay-Cee-L, Phosphate-Sandoz and Maalox.

What is the evidence for feeding patients with pancreatitis?

A 2004 *British Medical Journal* meta-analysis of parenteral nutrition versus enteral nutrition in patients with acute pancreatitis included six studies, which concluded that there were no significant differences in mortality or non-infectious complications between the two groups of patients.

Enteral nutrition should be the preferred route of nutritional support in patients with acute pancreatitis.

ABDOMINAL COMPARTMENT SYNDROME

What is abdominal compartment syndrome?

Definition

Abdominal compartment syndrome (ACS) is defined as a sustained IAP >20 mmHg associated with new organ dysfunction/failure.

What is intra-abdominal hypertension?

Intra-abdominal hypertension (IAH) is defined by a sustained or repeated IAP ≥12 mmHg.

What are the causes?

Causes of raised intra-abdominal pressure (IAP):
➤ retroperitoneal
➤ intraperitoneal
➤ oedema in necrotising pancreatitis
➤ haemorrhage
➤ pelvic haematoma
➤ visceral oedema
➤ retroperitoneal haematoma
➤ abdominal packing
➤ bleeding after aortic surgery
➤ bowel dilatation
➤ oedema related to resuscitation
➤ mesenteric venous obstruction
➤ pneumoperitoneum.

What patients are at risk for developing ACS?

At-risk patients:
➤ major trauma
➤ damage control surgery
➤ laparotomy for bleeding, ischaemia, etc.

➤ re-laparotomy for postoperative complications

➤ massive volume resuscitation.

What is the pathophysiology?

What are the effects of ACS?

➤ Gut and hepatic effects.

➤ Renal effects.

➤ Cardiovascular effects.

➤ Respiratory effects.

➤ CNS effects.

➤ Abdominal wall effects.

Gut and hepatic effects

Splanchnic and hepatic blood flow.

➤ Decreased mucosal blood flow.

➤ Flow in animal models with IAP >10 mmHg.

➤ Ischaemia at >40 mmHg.

➤ Gastric mucosal acidosis with IAP improves with decompression.

Renal effects

➤ IAP 15–20 mmHg renal blood flow.

➤ GFR with anuria when >30 mmHg.

➤ No effect of stenting.

➤ Parenchymal compression and renal vascular resistance.

Reversible by decompression.

Cardiovascular effects

Venous return by compression of IVC and portal vein.

➤ Intra-thoracic pressure, LV compliance, cardiac contractility and CO.

➤ Peripheral oxygen delivery.

➤ Increases SVR.

➤ Hypovolaemia.

Respiratory effects

Reduced airway compliance

➤ Elevation of diaphragm, thoracic volume and intra-thoracic pressure.

➤ Airway pressures to maintain ventilation.

➤ Atelectasis.

➤ V/Q mismatch.
➤ Hypoxia, hypercarbia, acidosis.

CNS effects
➤ Impaired venous return and cerebral pooling.
➤ Intra-cranial pressure (ICP).
➤ Decreased cerebral perfusion pressure.

How do you measure it?
Measurement of IAP
➤ Do NOT rely on physical examination.
➤ Direct measurement NOT advised.
➤ Indirect assessment of IAP by bladder pressure is gold standard.
➤ Several commercial kits available.
➤ Foley catheter in bladder.
➤ Manometric technique.
➤ Distance of fluid above pubic symphysis.
➤ IAP in cm H_2O (1 mmHg = 1.36 cm H_2O).
➤ U-tube technique.
➤ Revised intravesicle technique.
➤ Pressure transducer and 50 mL saline.

What are the principles of management?
➤ Serial monitoring of IAP.
➤ Improve abdominal wall compliance.
➤ Pain, agitation, sedation, paralysis (NMB).
➤ Optimisation of systemic and organ perfusion.
➤ Body positioning – supine better.
➤ Bowel decompression.
➤ NG tubes, enemata, prokinetic agents.
➤ Intra-abdominal drainage, e.g. collections.
➤ Correct positive fluid balance.
➤ Avoid overresuscitation.
➤ Diuretics.
➤ Surgical decompression for severe cases.

What is a damage control laparotomy?
A damage control laparotomy (DCL) is a laparotomy performed usually for trauma where the primary aim is to control haemorrhage and limit sepsis in the first instance. It is usually performed in an environment of hypothermia, acidosis, and coagulopathy and hence the priority is essentially to get the patient off the operating table as soon as possible. It should take no more than 45 minutes.

Essentially, there are three stages:
1 The initial laparotomy.

2   The ICU.

3   Definitive repair.

When would you consider doing a DCL?

The factors when a DCL should be considered are:

➤ unstable patient

➤ coagulapathy

➤ on escalating inotropes

➤ pH <7.1

➤ lactate >5.

How would you do a temporary abdominal closure (TAC)?

Wrap a large abdominal pack in sterile clear adhesive film dressing. Place this over the bowel. Place 2 × 24 fr suction drains on top of this first layer, entering from opposite side of the wound and not reaching below the fascia. Add a second film-wrapped abdominal pack to complete the 'sandwich'. Cover the whole dressing with a large clear film adhesive dressing.

This is air-tight and prevents leaks unlike older closure methods. The drains must be connected to suction and not in contact with abdominal contents.

Use this when after reduction the bowel lies higher than the fascial horizon.

POST OPERATIVE CARE

What are the causes of acute post-op confusion?

➤ Hypoxia (the most common cause).

➤ Electrolyte imbalance.

➤ Drugs, e.g. PCA, epidural, opiates.

➤ Alcohol (either withdrawal or ingestion).

➤ Infection.

➤ Haemorrhage.

How would you classify metabolic acidosis?

Metabolic acidosis may be defined as pH <7.35 with a base excess less than −2.

It may be classified according to the aetiology of whether there is excess acid or excess loss of bicarbonate.

Excess acid is typically associated with an increased anion gap and causes are:

➤ DKA

➤ uraemia

➤ ethylene glycol

➤ salicylates

➤ rhabdomyolysis

➤ lactic acidosis.

Loss of bicarbonate in a surgical patient is associated with a normal anion gap and causes are:

➤ diarrhoea
➤ fistula
➤ ileal conduit
➤ renal tubular acidosis
➤ ileostomy.

How would you calculate the anion gap and what is the normal value?
$(Na^+ + K^+) - (Cl^- - HCO_3^-)$
A normal value is 8–12.

KEY EMERGENCY SURGERY PROCEDURES
When would you use a caval filter?

I would follow the UK guidelines in the *British Journal of Haematology* (2006).

Indications

➤ Prevention of pulmonary embolism (PE) in patients with contraindication to warfarin.
➤ In pregnancy for those who have contraindication to warfarin (warfarin is teratogenic in the first trimester) or who develop extensive venous thrombolism (VTE) shortly before delivery.
➤ Should be considered in any pre-op patient with recent VTE in whom anticoagulation must be interrupted.

Complications

➤ Renal failure (renal vein occlusion).
➤ Misplacement.
➤ Pneumothorax.
➤ Haematoma.
➤ Air embolism.
➤ Carotid artery puncture.
➤ AV fistula.
➤ Recurrent DVT.
➤ IVC thrombosis.
➤ Post-phlebitic syndrome.
➤ Filter migration/filter fracture.
➤ Migration of guidewires.

How would you manage a 75-year-old female with strangulated femoral hernia?

➤ Full history and examination (vital signs, scars, lump, obstruction, PR, peritonitis).
➤ ABC/fluid balance.
➤ ABG/catheter.

➤ IVABs.
➤ DVT prophylaxis.
➤ Theatre.

How will you proceed in theatre?
➤ Supine position.
➤ Prep for full laparotomy.
➤ Modified McEvedy approach.
➤ Four fingerbreadths above pubic tubercle.
➤ External oblique divided.
➤ Rectus retracted medially and inferior epigastric vessels divided.
➤ Pre-peritoneal space developed and femoral canal exposed from above.

You are doing a laparoscopic appendix. What will you do if it is normal?

This depends on whether you find any other pathlogy or not. I think the safest and probably best practice is that if you find no other pathology within the abdomen then remove the appendix.

If you find something else, e.g. ovarian cyst, etc., then leave the appendix. This can be justified on the basis of a study from Nuneaton (Singhal *et al.* 2007) which showed that in the abscence of any other pathology a macroscopically normal-looking appendix may have microscopic inflammation in up to 10% cases.

Appendix mass or abscess?

This is almost a guaranteed question in the emergency viva. Be sure you have a clear strategy and be able to defend it. The management of acute appendicitis is an appendicectomy. Grumbling or chronic appendicitis does not exist. Missed appendicitis does exist.

An appendix mass typically will present with a longer history usually as a result of the delayed presentation. If the patient is well, then this is probably best managed conservatively and may well settle with antibiotics. If it is an older patient, then the concern is to avoid missing a caecal cancer and so the patient should have the large bowel imaged, such as either CT or barium enema after the acute event. In a younger age group the concern is Crohn's disease.

The examiner will then discuss interval appendicectomy. This is no longer justified, as 92% of cases that have resolved will no longer develop recurrent symptoms.

The appendix abscess on the other hand will probably require intervention, especially if there is rising WCC and swinging pyrexia. The options here are either percutaneous drainage or surgery. Again this is a clinical decision and a well patient getting better on antibiotics should be managed accordingly.

How would you manage a 12 year-old boy with acute unilateral scrotal pain?

This must be treated as acute testicular torsion until proven otherwise.

The differential diagnosis here may include:

➤ hydatid cyst of Morgagni
➤ epidydymo-orchitis
➤ idiopathic scrotal oedema.

The exam answer here is that unless you are absolutely certain that this is not a hydatid of Morgagni (which you can argue either way for operative treatment), then this patient warrents urgent scrotal exploration under GA in the next available theatre.

What are the causes of a psoas abscess?

➤ Crohn's disease.
➤ Diverticular disease.
➤ Appendicitis.
➤ Caecal carcinoma.
➤ Osteomyelitis.
➤ Spinal TB.
➤ Pancreatic abscess.
➤ Peri-nephric abscess.
➤ Infected pelvic haematoma.
➤ Staphylococcus sepsis.

What are the issues for managing a patient with acute appendicitis who has sickle cell anaemia?

A clinical diagnosis of acute appendicitis will require an urgent operation. Second, a sickle cell crisis itself may cause an acute abdomen, so it will be essential to make a correct diagnosis. Third, acute appendicitis causes fever, acidosis and an increased risk of sickling.

Key surgical issues

➤ Patient should have clinical and baseline investigations.
➤ Severity of sickle cell determined by Hb SS subtype.
➤ The complications of vaso-occlusive crisis cause organ infarction, poor spleen function and hepatosplenomegaly.
➤ The patient needs to be kept warm, well filled with adequate supplemental oxygen aiming for normothermia, avoiding hypoxemia, acidosis in order to minimise the risk of sickling.
➤ Narcotic analgesia will be required but hypoventilation will be a risk.
➤ More likely to require a blood transfusion if significant bloods loss.
➤ Senior surgeon to do procedure.

How would you manage a 16-year-old female with right iliac fossa pain?

Key surgical issues

➤ History and examination.
➤ Bloods.
➤ HCG.
➤ Clinical diagnosis of appendicitis.
➤ Ultrasound.
➤ Diagnostic laparoscopy.

A 24-year-old pregnant female presents with RIF pain. How would you assess and proceed?

➤ Ideally, admit to gynae in first instance to exclude ectopic.
➤ If appendicitis is clinically apparent, then laparoscopy is warranted.

Approximately 1 in 500 women will require non-obstetrical abdominal surgery during their pregnancy. The most common non-obstetrical surgical emergencies complicating pregnancy are acute appendicitis, cholecystitis and intestinal obstruction. Although foetal safety during diagnostic imaging is an important goal for surgeons and patients, the benefits to the mother outweigh the risk to the foetus, bearing in mind that the risk of foetal morbidity and mortality also increases when the mother is faced with an acute surgical emergency.

The following guidelines have been taken from SAGES regarding the diagnosis, treatment and use of laparoscopy during pregnancy.

Ultrasound imaging during pregnancy is safe and useful in identifying the cause of acute abdominal pain in the pregnant patient.

Expeditious and accurate diagnosis should take precedence over concerns for ionising radiation. Contemporary multi-detector CT rotocols deliver a radiation dose to the foetus below detrimental levels and may be considered as an appropriate test during pregnancy, depending on the clinical situation.

MRI can be performed at any stage of pregnancy without the use of IV gadolinium.

Intraoperative and endoscopic cholangiography exposes the mother and foetus to minimal radiation and may be used selectively during pregnancy. ERCP also has risks beyond the radiation exposure such as bleeding and pancreatitis. In non-pregnant patients, the risk of bleeding is 1% and the risk of pancreatitis is 3.5%.

Diagnostic laparoscopy is safe and effective when used in pregnancy. Several recent studies have shown that pregnant patients may indergo laparoscopic surgery safely during any trimester without any appreciated increased risk to the mother or foetus. It has also been suggested that delaying surgical intervention in patients with symptomatic gallstone disease during pregnancy may lead to further complications of gallstone diease such as acute cholecystitis and gallstone pancreatitis which can lead to higher spontaneous abortion rates and preterm labour.

Gravid patients should be placed in the left lateral position to minimise compression of the IVC and aorta.

Initial pneumoperitoneum can be safely obtained with either open, verress needle or optical trocar technique.

CO_2 insufflation pressure of 10–15 mmHg can be safely used for laparoscopy in pregnant patients.

Intraoperative and postoperative preumatic compression devices and early postoperative ambulation are recommended for DVT prophylaxis in the pregnant patient. There is no data regarding use of LMWH for prophylaxis in pregnant patients undergoing laparoscopy. It has been suggested that patients undergoing extended major surgery should have some.

Laparoscopic cholecystecomy is the treatment of choice in the pregnant patient with gallbladder disease regardless of trimester.

Laparoscopic appendicectomy may be performed safely in pregnant patients with clinical suspicion of appendicitis.

Foetal heart monitoring should occur pre- and postoperatively in the setting of urgent abdominal surgery during pregnancy.

How do you manage sigmoid volvulus?

A sigmoid volvulus rotates 180–720 degrees in EITHER direction.

It typically presents with pain, constipation and abdominal distension.

The typical AXR is below giving the classical 'coffee-bean' sign.

Decompress in theatre with a flexible sigmoidoscopy rather than a rigid, as:

➤ it will allow an accurate diagnosis
➤ you may exclude other pathologies
➤ you can directly inspect the mucosa

This will usually have a 90% success rate.

How would you manage an anastomotic leak following sigmoid colostomy?

➤ Resuscitate.
➤ ABC.
➤ Fluid balance.
➤ Review charts and urine output.
➤ Look at operation note.
➤ Clinical examination (peritonitis = laparotomy).
➤ Haematological investigations (bloods, X-match, ABG).
➤ Radiology (CXR, GGF enema, CT).
➤ Conservative options (IVABs, drainage).
➤ Surgical options (stoma +/– mucous fistula).

Key points
➤ Mean day 12.
➤ 35–45% are subclinical (radiological).
➤ >80% proceed to laparotomy.
➤ 70% end up with permanent stoma.
➤ Typically day 3–6.
➤ Temp, AF, BP, hiccoughs.
➤ Only 25% have peritonitis.

When do you operate in small bowel obstruction?

You may get an opening question on the causes of small bowel obstruction. A quick list to hand may be useful:
➤ adhesions
➤ hernias
➤ caecal pathology
➤ gallstone ileus
➤ foreign bodies/bezoars
➤ small bowel tumours
➤ Crohn's disease
➤ intussusception
➤ polyps
➤ radiation enteritis.

Clearly, adhesions are the most common cause of small bowel obstruction and you may get a scenario which you may have to operate. A useful paper published in the *British Journal of Surgery* (2010) showed that failure of oral contrast to reach the caecum within 4 hours, and certainly within 12 hours, suggests that surgical intervention is required.

Management of small bowel obstruction

A 75-year-old male is admitted with typical small bowel obstruction on AXR, with no hernias and no previous surgery. How will you proceed?

This is an examiners' favourite in that they want to test your decision-making ability to take a patient to theatre. You may choose to make an argument for getting a CT prior to surgery but unless the patient is clearly unfit for surgery, a laparotomy is the correct answer for this question.

At laparotomy, you find a large thickened mass of carcinomatosis with matted loops of dilated small bowel encasing the mesenteric vessles. A trial dissection is unhelpful. What will you do next?

Again here they are testing your ability to make a consultant decision. Options are to take a frozen section to get a diagnosis as either metastatic pancreatic adenocarcinoma or lymphoma may have different outcomes. A bypass procedure or venting gastrostomy may be further options. However, in the above scenario, it is unlikely that this is survivable and the correct decision is to close the abdomen and palliate the patient.

Toxic megacolon in a 40-year-old with acute colitis

Key principles revolve around perioperative management and the decision YOU are going to make about when and how to take the colon out.

➤ Daily bloods and clinical examination.
➤ Daily AXR (>6 cm diameter = toxic megacolon).
➤ Ideally should be joint care with GI physicians.
➤ IV steroids and fluid resuscitation.

Indications for surgery

➤ Generalised peritonitis.
➤ Free air under the diaphragm.
➤ Toxic colon on AXR.
➤ Failed medical treatment.

The Oxford study showed that if there were more than eight bowel motions per day and CRP >45 after 3 days of IV steroids, then there was an 85% chance of colectomy.

What can you tell me about pseudo-obstruction?

➤ Acute colonic pseudo-obstruction is characterised by clinical and radiological evidence of acute large bowel obstruction in the absence of a mechanical cause.
➤ The condition usually affects elderly people with underlying comorbidities.

Causes

Systemic causes:
➤ stroke
➤ myocardial infarction
➤ congestive heart failure
➤ electrolyte imbalance
➤ drug induced
➤ antidepressants
➤ opiates.

Infective causes:
➤ systemic sepsis
➤ herpes zoster infection
➤ pneumonia
➤ acute cholecystitis
➤ acute pancreatitis
➤ pelvic abscess.

Neurological causes:
➤ Parkinson's disease
➤ Alzheimer's disease.

Surgical causes:
➤ caesarean section
➤ gynaecological or pelvic surgery
➤ hip surgery
➤ mechanical ventilation
➤ spinal cord trauma
➤ pelvic trauma.

Management

Management strategy:
➤ NPO
➤ IV fluid replacement
➤ correction of electrolyte imbalances (K and Mg)
➤ rectal tube may occasionally be effective
➤ avoid drugs delaying gut motility (such as opiates, anticholinergics and calcium-channel blockers).

Osmotic laxatives, e.g. lactulose are contraindicated as they may promote colonic bacterial fermentation and produce gas.
➤ The limit of purely supportive measures cannot be stated exactly but in most situations should not exceed 48–72 hours.
➤ A duration of 6 days has been shown to lead to greater risk of complication.
➤ The exact 'at risk' caecal diameter is commonly cited to be 12 cm.

Pharmacological therapy:
➤ Intravenous neostigmine has been tested in controlled trials and remains the mainstay of treatment.
➤ Neostigmine is a reversible acetylcholinesterase inhibitor that increases the activation of muscarinic receptors by preventing the breakdown of acetylcholine, thus promoting colonicmotor activity and intestinal transit.
➤ Oral administration of neostigmine is not recommended because of its erratic absorption.
➤ Three placebo-controlled double-blind randomised trials have documented the effectiveness of neostigmine.
➤ One study recorded that 10 of 11 patients receiving the drug intravenously showed marked clinical and radiological improvement, compared with 10 patients in the placebo group who had no response (Ponce *et al.*).

Massive PR bleed on warfarin?

➤ ABC.
➤ IV access.
➤ Bloods and X-match 4 units.
➤ Clotting/INR.
➤ Indications for warfarin, e.g. AF vs mechanical valve.

Decisions

➤ Interventional radiology and embolisation.
➤ Shocked and failure to stop bleeding = surgery and correction of clotting (vitamin K, FFP, Octaplex).
➤ Location of blood loss – OGD if malaena.

Case scenario: A 65-year-old male on warfarin for AF is admitted with bleeding duodenal ulcer.

Surgical issues:
➤ surgery is essential
➤ high morbidity and mortality expected
➤ warfarin is safe to reverse as no metal valve present
➤ vitamin K
➤ FFP
➤ Octaplex (prothrombin complex concentrate).

Use of Octaplex™:
➤ for urgent correction of clotting factor deficiency
➤ more rapid-acting than FFP
➤ decreased risk of fluid overload
➤ decreased risk of analphylaxis
➤ decreased risk of viral transmission
➤ contains all four vitamin K-dependent factors.

Ischaemic bowel at laparotomy?

➤ Assess cause: embolic, AF?
➤ Assess extent: widespread/not survivable vs colon (= colectomy).
➤ Small bowel: limits of resection (short bowel syndrome, high output).

How would you manage a gallstone ileus?

A 65-year-old female patient with recurrent cholecystitis presents with andominal pain and vomiting. What radiological features would support diagnosis of cholecystoduodenal fistula?
➤ Pneumobilia.
➤ Small bowel obstruction.

This is usually a CT diagnosis and will require a laparotomy. Options at surgery are:

➤ milk the gallstone distally into the caecum
➤ proximal enterotomy and primary closure
➤ small bowel resection.

It may be wise to avoid a cholecystectomy at this laparotomy.

Pre-cordial stab wound in A&E

Must exclude cardiac tamponade!

May well have simple open pneumothorax but features of tamponade must be looked for and excluded. This question puts you in the scenario of a peri-arrest patient typically with a blood pressure of 60 mmHg, impending tamponade and no cardiothoracic surgeon available.

Although ATLS teaches pericardiocentesis, it will not work and the patient in extremis is likely to succumb. The only possible solution is an emergency thoracotomy, ideally in an operating theatre but if the patient is about to arrest then this will have to be done in resus.

A general surgeon should be able to do this and may be so expected. This has been asked before in the exit exam. The definitive surgical trauma skills (DSTS) course provides excellent preparation for this rare emergency. The key manoeuvres are:

➤ The patient must be intubated.
➤ Open the left chest between the fifth and sixth interspace with a 23-blade scalpel.
➤ Cut through the intercostal muscles with a pair of Mayo scissors. (Steps 2–3 should take no more than 30 seconds.)
➤ Insert a Finochietto rib-spreader (the correct way round).
➤ Incise the parietal pleura with scissors and clamp the descending thoracic aorta.
➤ Incise the pericardium vertically avoiding the phrenic nerves that run down the lateral sides of the heart.
➤ At this point you hopefully can find a single chamber stab wound and suture it. Temporary control may be obtained with a Foley catheter.

Stab wound to RUQ – patient unstable

Typical exam question here is: a 40-year-old male presents with a knife wound to the right upper quadrant and BP 60/40 despite 2 units of blood. How would you proceed?

The exam answer and key principles are:

➤ prepare for theatre (X-match blood)
➤ midline laparotomy incision
➤ four-quadrant packing
➤ Pringle manoeuvre
➤ packing of liver (leave packs in for 36–48 hours)
➤ ITU.

This scenario will inevitably lead on to discussion of the lethal triad, management of coagulopathy, use of blood products, temporary abdominal closure and the abdominal compartment syndrome.

Patient has sustained a penetrating knife injury to the right flank and is unstable. Urgent laparotomy is performed revealing laceration to IVC. Proceed?

➤ Midline incision.
➤ Four-quadrant packing.
➤ Right medial visceral rotation (Cattell-Brasch manoeuvre).
➤ Proximal and distal control.
➤ Foley catheter.
➤ Direct repair 3/0 Prolene.

DIATHERMY
How does diathermy work?

In monopolar diathermy, the surgeon uses an active electrode with a small surface area tip to concentrate a powerful current producing heat at the operative site. The large return electrode plate which completes the circuit spreads the current over a wide area, so that it is less concentrated and it produces little heat.

In bipolar diathermy, the current occurs between two small active electrodes.

Surgical diathermy uses either a cutting or a coagulation mode. Cutting occurs when sufficient heat is applied to tissue to cause cell water to vapourise into steam. In this cutting mode the current is a continous wave form. In the COAG form, there is an interrupted waveform with the current.

MISCELLANEOUS VIVA QUESTIONS

The following are a set of random exam viva questions that have been asked in the past. I have not given any answers with them. They are there to give you scenarios that you may find yourself in, both while on-call and in the exam. Hopefully they can be used as topics for discussion with your colleagues in the weeks prior to the exam.

➤ A knife is inserted into the rectum during an assault in Glasgow. How do you proceed?
➤ How do you approach bladder rupture?
➤ How do you perform an emergency thoracotomy?
➤ A 75-year-old man presents with AF, mid-gut pain and rectal bleeding. How do you proceed?
➤ Your speciality trainee gets a needle stick injury. What is your next step?
➤ A patient presents with free air under diaphragm. How will you proceed?
➤ At laparoscopy for RIF pain you find acute Crohn's disease. How will you proceed?

➤ A 10-year-old female patient 5 days post lap-appendix fails to settle. Discuss.
➤ What are the NICE guidelines for head injuries?
➤ How would you manage a 42-year-old female with recurrent biliary colic on warfarin for previous DVT?

PART TWO

MCQs and SBAs

1 Which of the following statements about gentamycin is INCORRECT?
   A It acts by inhibiting the 50S ribosome
   B It acts by decreasing protein synthesis via mRNA
   C It should be avoided in myasthenia gravis
   D It can be given once daily in a dose of 7 mg/kg
   E It can cause both ototoxicity and nephrotoxicity

2 Which of the following is the cause of an INCREASED anion gap?
   A Hypercalcaemia
   B Hypermagnesaemia
   C Lithium toxicity
   D Hypoalbuminaemia
   E Ethylene glycol ingestion

3 A 22-year-old male sustains a pre-cordial stab wound: BP 60/40, pulse 140 and has distended neck veins. Immediate treatment might include:
   A Sub-xiphoid pericardiocentesis
   B 2 litres normal saline IV
   C Needle decompression in second intercostal space mid-clavicular line
   D Emergency thoracotomy and cross clamp aorta
   E All of the above

4 Which of the following does NOT require a duplex scan prior to surgery?
   A Primary long saphenous vein surgery
   B Primary short saphenous vein ligation
   C Recurrent long saphenous vein surgery
   D Recurrent short saphenous vein surgery
   E Surgery for chronic venous insufficiency

5 Which of the following does NOT cause a metabolic alkalosis?
   A Vomiting
   B Pyloric stenosis
   C Hypokalaemia
   D Frusemide
   E Spironolactone

6 Which of the following is NOT a feature of disseminated intravascular coagulation (DIC)?
   A Increased fibrin degradation products (FDPs)
   B Thrombocytopenia
   C Increased prothrombin time (PT)
   D Negative D-dimer
   E Schistocytes on blood film

7 Which of the following statements regarding haemophilia A is TRUE?
   A Factor-IX deficiency
   B Autosomal dominant inheritance
   C Occurs in 1 in 1000 people
   D It is also called Christmas disease
   E Causes an increased APTT

8 Which of the following statements regarding von Willebrand's disease is TRUE?
   A Occurs in 1 in 1000 people
   B Is 4 times more common in females
   C Typically has raised prothrombin time (PT)
   D Thrombocytopenia is common
   E APTT is usually normal

9 Which of the following statements regarding paragangliomas is CORRECT?
   A They are usually malignant
   B They are derived from chromaffin-positive neural cells
   C Are associated with MEN 2A and MEN 2B
   D 90% occur in the head and neck and are known as chemodectomas
   E Are typically painful swellings

10 Which of the following statements regarding *Clostridium difficile* is INCORRECT?
   A It is a Gram-negative anaerobic organism
   B It is a normal gut commensal in most children
   C Omeprazole is a risk factor for development
   D Is sensitive to Linezolid
   E Produces an enterotoxin and a cytotoxin

11   The commonest cause of death following fractured neck of femur is:
   A   Bronchopneumonia
   B   Left ventricular failure
   C   Myocardial infarction
   D   Stroke
   E   Pulmonary embolism

12   Which of the following is the most common predisposing factor for developing necrotising fasciitis?
   A   Immunosuppression
   B   Malnutrition
   C   Steroids
   D   Diabetes
   E   IV drug abuse

13   Which of the following statements regarding popliteal artery aneurysms is FALSE?
   A   They are the most common peripheral aneurysm
   B   50% are bilateral
   C   40% are associated with AAA
   D   They should be repaired if >2 cm
   E   They typically present with rupture and shock

14   Which of the following is NOT a component of the IMRIE scoring system for pancreatitis?
   A   Age
   B   Calcium
   C pO_2
   D   Creatinine
   E   Albulmin

15   A patient has developed a liver abscess secondary to acute cholecystitis. The most likely organism is:
   A   *E. coli*
   B   *Strep. milleri*
   C   *Strep. pneumonia*
   D   *Staphlococcus aureus*
   E   *Listeria monocytogenes*

16   What organism is most commonly responsible for the development of gas gangrene?
   A   *Clostridium welchi*
   B   *Clostridium septicum*
   C   *Clostridium perfringens*
   D   *Clostridium tetani*
   E   *Streptococcus pyogenes*

17 Which of the following is NOT a boundary of the ischio-rectal fossa?
   A External anal sphincter
   B Obturator internus
   C Levator ani
   D Anal skin
   E Ischial tuberosity

18 Which of the following options is NOT a branch of the trigeminal nerve?
   A Supraorbital
   B Supratrochlear
   C Maxillary
   D Infraorbital
   E Buccal

19 Which of the following structures does NOT run through the carpal tunnel?
   A Median nerve
   B Flexor pollicis longus
   C Flexor digitorum superficialis
   D Flexor digitorum profundus
   E Palmaris longus

20 Which of the following nerves does NOT arise from the posterior cord of the brachial plexus?
   A Radial nerve
   B Axillary nerve
   C Ulnar nerve
   D Thoracodorsal
   E Upper subscapular nerve

21 Which of the following arteries do NOT arise from the subclavian artery?
   A Vertebral
   B Internal mammary
   C Internal thoracic
   D Superior thyroid
   E Inferior thyroid

22 Which of the following statements regarding Gilbert's syndrome is TRUE?
   A It is more common in females
   B It is X-linked
   C Typically causes an obstructive pattern on liver function tests
   D Causes an increase in unconjugated bilirubin levels
   E Causes post-hepatic jaundice

23   Which of the following bacteria is Gram-positive?
   A   *E. coli*
   B   *Klebsiella*
   C   *H. pylori*
   D   *C. difficile*
   E   *Proteus mirabilis*

24   A man develops pyrexia, tachycardia and lower abdominal pain on day 6, post sigmoid colectomy. What is the most likely diagnosis?
   A   Cellulitis
   B   Myocardial infarction
   C   Anastomotic leak
   D   UTI
   E   Pneumonia

25   Which of the following would cause the oxy-haemoglobin dissociation curve to shift to the LEFT?
   A   Hypercapnia
   B   Increased 2,3-DPG
   C   High altitude
   D   Pregnancy
   E   Increased pH

26   Which of the following is a recognised cause of hypercalcaemia?
   A   Hypoalbulminaemia
   B   Alkalosis
   C   Vitamin D deficiency
   D   Sarcoidosis
   E   Pancreatitis

27   Which of the following is NOT a component of the Truelove-Witts classification for acute colitis?
   A   Passage of >6 stools per day
   B   White cell count >20
   C   Fever >37.5 °C
   D   Anaemia <10.5 g/dL
   E   ESR >30

28   Which of the following is a pure vasoconstrictor?
   A   Dopamine
   B   Adrenaline
   C   Noradrenaline
   D   Milrinone
   E   Dobutamine

29 A 42-year-old renal patient has a brachio-basilic fistula made 3 months ago. He now has arm claudication and the tips of his fingers have become necrotic. What is the likely pathology here?
   A Infected graft
   B Stenosis
   C Steal phenomenon
   D Raynaud's syndrome
   E Embolisation

30 A 65-year-old male has a 6 cm infra-renal abdominal aortic aneurysm. The neck is 15 mm with a 40-degree angulation with respect to the longitudinal axis. There is iliac involvement. Which of the following is the most suitable?
   A Open repair
   B Conservative management
   C Surveillance scan in 6 months
   D EVAR
   E Axillo-bifem bypass

31 A man has a reversed LSV fem-pop bypass for disabling claudication. Initially, post operation, the graft is working but goes down on day 2. What is the most common reason for graft failure?
   A Technical failure
   B Superficial wound haematoma
   C Systemic atherosclerosis
   D Smoking
   E Poor diabetic control

32 A 75-year-old male has a 6 cm AAA. He is due for elective repair but is found to have MRSA on swabs from nose and skin. What would you do?
   A Proceed with surgery
   B Cancel and erradicate
   C Proceed with surgery under antibiotic cover
   D Repeat swabs
   E Treat with IV vancomycin and proceed with surgery

33 A 45-year-old male is in theatre for a laparoscopic appendix that is converted to open because of a large tumour of the right colon encasing R-ureter and kidney. There is no obvious liver metastasis. What is the most appropriate next step?
   A Ileocolic bypass
   B On table IVP to assess function of the left kidney
   C Shave tumour off kidney and ureter
   D Proceed with right hemicolectomy and radical nephrectomy
   E Stent the ureters and proceed with right hemicolectomy

34 An 85-year-old with dementia, COPD, and severe peripheral vascular disease presents with a 7 cm full thickness rectal prolapse. What is the most appropriate management?
   A Conservative medical Rx
   B Delorme's procedure
   C Laparoscopic rectopexy
   D Altemeire's procedure
   E Open resection/rectopexy
   F STARR procedure

35 Which of the following are considered essential steps in a TME?
   A division of Waldeyer's fascia
   B Posterior dissection in recto-sacral plane
   C Ligation of lateral ligaments
   D High tie IMA
   E Division of space posterior to Denonvilliers' fascia

36 A man has had a below-knee amputation 6 weeks with a non-healing stump. What organism is most likely responsible?
   A Methicillin-resistant *Staphylococcus aureus* (MRSA)
   B Methicillin-sensitive *Staphylococcus aureus* (MSSA)
   C *Klebsilla*
   D *E. coli*
   E *Bacteroides*

37 A 4-year-old boy 1-week post open appendicectomy presents with a non-tender mass in the RIF. He is apyrexial and has a normal WCC. How do you proceed?
   A Discharge home
   B PO antibiotics
   C Observe for 24 hours
   D Laparotomy
   E CT

38 A 40-year-old male sustains a penetrating stab wound to his left chest. You are called to A&E resus. He was initially unstable but has responded to fluids. An ICD yields 1200 mL initially, then stops and his vital signs stabilise. The most appropriate next step is?
   A Thoracotomy
   B Median sternotomy
   C ITU and blood transfusion
   D CT scan
   E FAST scan

39 A 55-year-old man has been endoscoped and has confirmed Barrett's oesophagus with high-grade dysplasia by two pathologists. What is the recommended treatment?
   A Treat with a 3-month course of proton pump inhibitor
   B Oesophajectomy
   C Repeat endoscopy and biopsy in 2 years
   D Aspirin and omeprazole
   E Surveillance endoscopy in 3 months

40 A patient is being staged for an oesophageal cancer at the OG junction 3 cm, and CT confirms coeliac node involvement with no other signs of distant metastasis. The correct staging is?
   A T2 N2 MO
   B T2 N2 M1
   C T2 N1 MO
   D T2 N1 M1
   E T2 N3 MO

41 A 55-year-old male in HDU is day 3 post anterior resection. His monitor shows a tachycardia of 120 with no P waves on the ECG. What should the first-line treatment be?
   A IV Digoxin
   B IV Amiodarone
   C IV Metoprolol
   D Carotid sinus massage
   E Adenosine

42 A 22-year-old male sustains a head injury in an assault. He opens his eyes to speech, makes groaning noises and localises to painful stimuli. His Glasgow coma scale (GCS) is?
   A 8
   B 9
   C 10
   D 11
   E 12

43 Which of the following has the least incidence of malignancy?
   A Insulinoma
   B Gastrinoma
   C VIPoma
   D Glucagonoma

44 Which of the following drugs is the most likely to cause avascular necrosis of the femur in a transplant patient?
A Tacrolimus
B OKT3
C Sirolimus
D Prednisolone
E Azathioprine

45 Which of the following is NOT required to diagnose brain stem death?
A Fixed and dilated pupils
B EEG
C A consultant
D CT scan
E A doctor of at least 5 years post-registration experience

46 What is the most reliable feature for an achalasia diagnosis?
A High-pressure contractions of oesophagus
B Manometry findings of aperistalsis
C High pressure LOS and failure of relaxation of LOS
D History
E Endoscopic findings

47 A female patient is recovering 2 days following a normal vaginal delivery. She collapses on the ward: BP 80/40 and pulse 120. Urgent blood gas shows base excess −6, pO_2 10 kPa, pCO_2 4.2 kPa, haemoglobin 6. There are no external signs of bleeding. The most likely cause is:
A Ruptured uterus
B Retained products of conception
C Ruptured splenic artery aneurysm
D Massive pulmonary embolism
E Septic shock

48 The most common presenting feature/s of a choledochal cyst is/are:
A Pain
B Jaundice
C Mass
D Pain and jaundice
E Jaundice and mass

49 What is the most appropriate method of feeding for a high output fistula following small bowel resection?
A Oral
B NG
C TPN
D PEG
E Jejunal

50 Which of the following are contraindications to PICC line insertion?
   A Infection
   B Thrombophlebitis
   C Abnormal clotting
   D Hypotension
   E Hypokalaemia

51 What is the most likely complication post central line insertion in a patient who presents with hypotension and abnormal heart sounds 12 hours following central line insertion?
   A Tension pneumothorax
   B Pneumothorax
   C Haemothorax
   D Mitral valve puncture
   E Air embolism

52 The oxyhaemoglobin dissociation curve is shifted to the left by:
   A A fall in pH
   B Foetal haemoglobin
   C Increased body temperature
   D Increased PCO_2
   E Increased 2,3-diphosphoglycerate

53 A 60-year-old female presenting jaundice with deranged LFTs, dilated CBD on US, no gallstones, MRCP shows no evidence of gallstones but CBD dilated. What is the next investigation?
   A Repeat MRI
   B CT
   C Liver biopsy
   D EUS
   E ERCP

54 A 75-year-old female has a GIST tumour with pelvic metastasis. What are the options for treatment?
   A Glivec
   B Octreotide
   C Surgery
   D Radiotherapy
   E Chemotherapy

55 A 65-year-old male presents with a massive haematemesis. Urgent endoscopy shows varices. What is the first-line therapeutic manoeuvre according to BSG guidelines?
A Phenol injection
B Stent
C Endoscopic banding
D Adrenaline injection
E Endoclips

56 Laparoscopic donor nephrectomy is superior to open nephrectomy for which one of the following reasons?
A Reduced incidence of complications in the recipient operation
B Reduced intraoperative blood loss
C Reduced postoperative analgesic requirements
D Reduced warm ischaemic time
E Shorter operating time

57 Abdominal compartment syndrome is associated with which of the following physiological parameters?
A Decrease venous return
B Decreased ICP
C Hypertension
D Bradycardia
E Increased renal blood flow

58 A 64-year-old man undergoes open right hemicolectomy for cancer. On his first postoperative day his BP is 100/50, pulse 90, CVP 4 with urine output of 15 mL/hr. What is the most appropriate next step?
A 250 mL Gelofusine
B Frusemide 40 mg IV
C Metaraminol infusion
D Normal saline 125 mL/hr
E Dopamine infusion

59 A 45-year-old female is recovering 2 days post total thyroidectomy. She develops peri-oral paraesthesia and her calcium is 1.8 mmol/L. How should this be treated?
A Oral calcium
B Oral vitamin D
C IV 10% calcium gluconate
D IV 10% calcium chloride
E Calcitonin

60 A patient on the evening following total thyroidectomy develops neck haematoma and stridor on ward. What do you do?
  A Remove clips
  B Remove clips AND open strap muscle layer
  C Urgent endotracheal intubation
  D Emergency cricothyroidotomy
  E Immediate return to theatre

61 Which of the following are features of Cushing's syndrome?
  A Hyperkalaemia
  B Weakness
  C Hypertension
  D Hair loss
  E Bradycardia

62 Which of the following are features of Conn's syndrome?
  A Hyperkalaemia
  B Polyuria
  C Oliguria
  D Hypertension
  E Hyponatraemia

63 A man undergoes a laparotomy for anastomotic leak post sigmoid colectomy. What is the most appropriate operation that should be done?
  A Laparoscopic washout
  B Washout and drain
  C Primary repair of leak
  D Hartmann's
  E Subtotal colectomy

64 A 15-year-old boy has a blunt abdominal trauma from a handlebar injury. What is injured?
  A Pancreas
  B Rectus sheath haematoma
  C Para-duodenal haematoma
  D Small bowel
  E Right lobe of liver

65 Histopathology unexpectedly reports a 1 cm carcinoid lesion resected from base of an appendix with clear margins. How would you proceed?
  A Discharge
  B Annual CT
  C Right hemicolectomy
  D 5-yearly CT
  E Annual colonoscopy

66 Everyone in a surgical unit (patient and staff) has diarrhoea and vomit-
    ting. What is the likely cause?
    A Norovirus
    B MRSA
    C *C. difficile*
    D *E. coli*

67 A 70-year-old man develops hypotension and sweating with associated
    abdominal pain 7 days post sigmoid colectomy. His temperature is 39 °C
    and WCC is 18. What is the most likely diagnosis?
    A Acute pyelonephritis
    B Anastmotic leak
    C Leaking AAA
    D Myocardial infarction
    E Pulmonary embolism

68 A 5-year-old child with known bronchiectasis is referred with an inguinal
    hernia. What is the most common cause of bronchiectasis in children?
    A Chronic aspiration
    B Congenital alpha-1-antitrypsin deficiency
    C Cystic fibrosis
    D Immunodeficiency disorders
    E Retained foreign bodies

69 What is the maximum permissible dose for plain bupivacaine in a child?
    A 2 mg/kg
    B 4 mg/kg
    C 6 mg/kg
    D 8 mg/kg
    E 10 mg/kg

70 Which of the following is NOT an essential part of a good patient-based
    functional outcome measure?
    A Consistency
    B Contestability
    C Reproducibility
    D Sensitivity to change
    E Validity

71 A 2-year-old child presents with a 5-day history of abdominal pain and vomiting with a confirmed intussuscepting. The mother states the child has lost 2kg in weight over the past week. What is the fluid deficit in mL?

A 120

B 240

C 1100

D 2000

E 3100

72 A 2-week-old term neonate is undergoing repair of a congenital diaphragmatic hernia. At induction of anaesthesis prior to repair, the child suddenly becomes difficult to ventilate despite a well-placed endothacheal tube. What condition must be excluded?

A Acute gastric volvulus

B Midgut volvulus

C Pulmonary embolism

D Pulmonary hypertensive crisis

E Tension pneumothorax

73 Conditions that may mimic symptoms of an MI are:

A Ruptured oesophagus

B Perforated duodenal ulcer

C Gastroesophageal reflux disorder

D Pulmonary embolism

E All of the above

74 Adenosine:

A Has a half-life of 30 minutes

B Should be avoided in patients with asthma

C Is active orally

D Must be given by slow IV infusion through a large peripheral vein

E Is chemically similar to adrenaline

75 Tetralogy of Fallot is characterised by:

A Atrial septal defects

B Left ventricular hypertrophy

C Pulmonary stenosis

D Patent ductus arteriosus

E Overriding of the pulmonary trunk

76 A farmer presents chest infection. What organism is the most likely cause?

A *Aspergillus fumigatum*

B *Candida albicans*

C *Pseudomonas*

D *Staphylococcus aureus*

E *E. coli*

77 An 18-year-old female presents with a swollen leg. There is no DVT. What is the likely diagnosis?
   A Lymphoedema precox
   B Elephantiasis
   C Lymphoedema tarde
   D Milroy's disease

78 A 75-year-old male with known vascular disease presents with rest pain in little toe. There is non-reconstructable disease? What is the best treatment option?
   A Analgesia
   B Below knee amputation
   C Amputate little toe
   D Analgesia
   E Thrombolysis

79 Which of the following statements about Li-Fraumeni syndrome is CORRECT?
   A It is autosomal recessive
   B It is caused by a mutation of the p53 suppressor gene
   C It is always associated with sarcomas
   D Having a first-degree relative with any cancer >45 years is diagnostic
   E It is more common in males

80 Which of the following statements about Paget's disease of the nipple is TRUE?
   A It requires a core biopsy for diagnosis
   B Definitive treatment is a mastectomy
   C 50% of patients will have an underlying malignancy
   D Accounts for 10% of breast cancers
   E Can be detected on a mammogram

81 Which of the following is NOT part of the criteria for NHS breast screening?
   A 50–70 years
   B 3 yearly-screenings
   C Single view
   D Females only

82 A 35-year-old female has a 2 cm breast lump. The core biopsy shows phyloides. What procedure should be followed?
   A WLE
   B Mastectomy
   C SLNB
   D Local excision

83 A 10-year-old male has PR bleeding for 3 months. There is no family history. A colonoscopy shows more than 60 polyps. What is the next step?
   A Repeat colonoscopy in 6 months
   B Await biopsy
   C Gastroscopy
   D Panproctocolectomy
   E Flexible sigmoidoscopy in 6 months

84 A 55-year-old presents with rectal bleeding with previous normal colonoscopy following previous colonoscopy with several 1 cm polyps. What is the next scoping interval if colonoscopy normal?
   A 1 year
   B 3 years
   C 5 years
   D 10 years
   E Discharge

85 A 20-year-old has a colonoscopy for Peutz-Jeghers. This is normal. What is the follow-up?
   A 6 months
   B 1 year
   C 2 years
   D 3 years
   E 5 years

86 A 65-year-old man undergoes a right hemicolectomy for Dukes' B adenocarcinoma. When should his next colonoscopy be performed?
   A 6 months
   B 1 year
   C 3 years
   D 5 years
   E 10 years

87 What are the common presenting complaints of thoracic outlet syndrome?
   A Median nerve compression
   B Ulnar nerve compression
   C Facial oedema
   D Swollen arm
   E Horner's syndrome

88 A 38-year-old female presents with a lump in the groin 4/52 post partum. The lump is present when standing. What is the likely cause?
A Saphena varix
B Femoral hernia
C Lymph node
D Inguinal hernia
E Femoral artery aneurysm

89 You are called to gynae theatre. You perform a laparoscopy and find a caecal mass plus peritoneal lesions. What do you do?
A Biopsy the mass
B Biopsy the mass and peritoneal lesion
C Arrange a CT
D Perform a right hemicolectomy
E Arrange urgent colonoscopy

90 A 70-year-old male with known peripheral vascular disease and intermittent claudication, previously documented SFA occlusion but good distal run-off, presents with critical ischaemic leg with tense calf and fixed mottling to knee. What is the most appropriate option?
A BKA
B AKA
C Thrombolysis
D Reversed LSV fem-pop
E Reversed PTFE fem-pop

91 Which of the following is NOT a pathological feature of Crohn's disease?
A Skip lesions
B Transmural ulceration
C Cobblestone appearance
D Crypt abscess
E Granulomata

92 An 85-year-old female is recovering in an orthopaedic ward following hemiarthroplasy after fractured neck of femur. She has abdominal pain and distension. What is the likely cause?
A Obstructing caecal cancer
B Ileus
C Pseudo-obstruction
D Sigmoid volvulus
E Small bowel obstruction

93 What is the first-line medical management for faecal incontinence?
   A Imodium
   B Biofeedback
   C Movicol
   D Lactulose
   E Amitriptyline

94 An 85-year-old female has a 1 cm Grade 3 invasive cancer removed while under local anaesthetic. The pathology is ER negative and HER-2 positive. There is no distant metastasis. Lymph nodes are clear. What is the most appropriate adjuvant treatment?
   A Tamoxifen
   B Exemstane
   C Anastrazole
   D Letrazole
   E Herceptin

95 Which of the following are pathological features likely to progress to invasive breast cancer?
   A Atypical hyperplasia
   B Apocrine metaplasia
   C Sclerosing adenosis
   D Endometrial hyperplasia
   E Atypical metaplasia

96 A 36-year-old female in the first trimester of pregnancy presents with a breast lump. Which of the following is the most appropriate investigation?
   A Mammogram
   B FNAC
   C Core biopsy
   D Stereotactic core
   E MRI

97 A 55-year-old female with previous mastectomy is having an elective cholecystectomy and develops urinary retention post-op. What is the likely cause?
   A Epidural-related retention
   B Spinal cord compression
   C Drug induced
   D Autonomic neuropathy
   E BPH

98 A 60-year-old male presents with absolute dysphagia 6 days after eating fish, when he developed pain in the left side of his neck. What is the diagnosis?
   A Oesophageal perforation
   B Oesophageal pouch
   C Oesophageal stricture
   D Laryngospasm
   E Oesophageal web

99 A patient has obstructive jaundice with previous Billroth II. What is the investigation of choice?
   A US
   B CT
   C ERCP
   D MRCP
   E EUS

100 An elderly man presents with haematemesis and chest pain. He has a known para-oesophageal hiatus hernia. What is the likely cause?
   A Myocardial infarction
   B AAA
   C Para-oesophageal volvulus
   D Boerhaave's syndrome
   E Perforated DU

101 What is the most common side-effect of foam injection of varicose veins?
   A Skin discoloration
   B Allergy
   C Analphylaxis
   D Stroke
   E Amourosis fugax

102 The single absolute indication for IVC filter placement is:
   A Recurrent PE on warfarin
   B DVT
   C PE
   D Duodenal ulcer
   E Atrial fibrillation

103 A patient is hypocalcaemic post thyroidectomy. What is the most appropriate medical treatment in an asymptomatic patient?
   A IV calcium chloride
   B IV calcium gluconate
   C Oral calcium and vitamin D
   D Calcitonin
   E Resonium

104 An elderly lady with known metastatic breast cancer is admitted dehydrated with a calcium level of 3.5 mmol/L. The most appropriate first-line treatment is:
A IV fluid resuscitation
B IV calcitonin
C IV pamidronate
D Resonium
E 5% dextrose

105 The overall responsibility for clinical governance in the hospital lies with the:
A GP
B Consultant
C Medical director
D Chief executive

106 A schizophrenic post appendectomy patient said he going to 'kill my wife'. He was seen by psychiatry and discharged. What will you do?
A Discharge
B Discharge and tell GP
C Tell wife and social worker
D Phone police and take advice

107 A patient is referred from a GUM clinic with anorectal ulceration. What is the likely infection?
A Gonorrhoea
B Chylamydia
C *Treponema pallidum* (Syphilis)
D AIDS
E Herpes

108 Which of the following is NOT a side-effect of statin?
A Myositis
B Nausea and vomiting
C Deranged LFTs
D Renal impairment
E Diarrhoea

109 What is the best feeding option for a patient 6 days post whipples with a 500 mL/day chyle leak in an abdominal drain with ascites and a feeding jejunostomy in situ?
A TPN
B Surgery
C NG feeding
D Jejunal feeding
E Oral intake

110 Which of the following antibiotics are effective against penicillinase-producing organisms?
   A Augmentin
   B Flucloxacillin
   C Ampicillin
   D Amocycillin
   E Penicillin V

111 Antibiotic prophylaxis is recommended for which of the following surgical procedures?
   A Open mesh repair inguinal hernia
   B TEP repair inguinal hernia
   C Vasectomy
   D Right hemicolectomy
   E Laparoscopic cholecystectomy

112 Which of the following antibiotics should be avoided in renal impairment?
   A Augmentin
   B Ciproxin
   C Flagyl
   D Gentamycin
   E Flucloxacillin

113 Which of the following is a common cause of gynaecomastia?
   A Antidepressants
   B Spironolactone
   C Hypothyroidism
   D Aspirin
   E Ranitidine

114 Regarding the gallbladder, which of the following statements is true?
   A The cystic duct is normally 5–6 cm long
   B The IVC is the anterior border of the foramen of windslow
   C The right hepatic artery crosses behind the common hepatic duct in 25% of cases
   D Normally holds about 250 mL of bile
   E The right hepatic artery usually gives off the cystic artery

115 Which of the following is NOT a feature of MEN-1 syndrome?
   A Zollinger-Ellison syndrome
   B Wermer's syndrome
   C Sipple's syndrome
   D Pituitary tumours
   E Hyperparathyroidism

116 Which of the following is a boundary of the femoral triangle?
   A   Lateral border of sartorius
   B   Pectineus
   C   Inguinal ligament
   D   Medial border of adductor magnus
   E   Medial border of gracilis

117 Which nerve mediates the cremasteric reflex?
   A   Ilioinguinal nerve
   B   Iliohypogastric nerve
   C   Obturator nerve
   D   Femoral nerve
   E   Genitofemoral nerve

118 Hyperamylasaemia may occur in all of the following conditions EXCEPT:
   A   Mumps
   B   Pancreatic carcinoma
   C   Ischaemic gut
   D   Ruptured AAA
   E   Diverticulitis

119 Which of the following is NOT a risk factor for ERCP-induced acute pancreatitis?
   A   Female
   B   Sphincter of oddi dysfunction
   C   >70 years
   D   Recurrent pancreatitis
   E   Jaundice

120 Carcinoid tumours are most commonly found in the:
   A   Stomach
   B   Small bowel
   C   Appendix
   D   Colon
   E   Duodenum

ANSWERS

1 **A.** Gentamycin is an aminoglycoside that acts by inhibiting the 30S ribosome.

2 **E.** Diabetic ketoacidosis (DKA), uraemia, ethylene glycol and aspirin overdose all cause an increased anion gap. All the others in this question cause a decreased anion gap.

3 **E.** All these may be required in this scenario.

4 **A.** This question appeared in a real FRCS exam.

5 **E.** All the others are well-recognised causes of metabolic alkalosis.

6 **D.** DIC associated with positive D-dimers.

7 **E.** Haemophilia A is associated with Factor-VIII deficiency. It is X-linked and occurs in approx. 1 in 10 000. Haemophilia B is known as Christmas disease.

8 **E.** Von Willebrand's disease occurs in 1% of the population, has an equal sex distribution. Clotting is usually normal and is treated with DDAVP prior to surgery in susceptible cases.

9 **C.** Paragangliomas are 97% benign and are derived from chromaffin-negative cells from the embryologically derived neural crest. They are usually painless masses and associated with both MEN 2A and 2B.

10 **A.** *C. diff* is a Gram-positive anaerobic organism and a normal gut commensal in about 70% children. Risks factors for infection are broad-spectrum antibiotic use, omeprazole use, ITU stay, burns patients and nursing home residents. It produces two toxins and is sensitive to oral vancomycin, IV or oral metronidazole, and linezolid.

11 **A.** Thirty per cent of all cases according to national mortality figures.

12 **D.** Diabetes mellitus is the most common predisposing factor.

13 **E.** Rupture is rare.

14 **D.**

15 **B.**

16 **C.**

17 **E.**

18 **E.** The trigeminal nerve has three main branches, the ophthalmic V1, the maxillary V2 and the mandibular V3. V1 has lacrimal, nasociliary and frontal branches (supraorbital and supratrochlear). The infraorbital branch comes off the maxillary. The mandibular has an anterior and posterior division (lingual and inferior alveolar). The buccal is a branch of the facial nerve.

19 **E.** The ulnar artery and nerve, the palmer branch of the median nerve and the Palmaris longus tendon all run superficial to the flexor retinaculum.

20 **C.** The five main nerves that arise from the posterior cord of the brachial plexus are the radial, axillary, thoracodorsal, upper subscapular and lower subscapular nerves.

21 **D.** The superior thyroid comes off the external carotid. All the others arise from the first part of the subclavian. The internal mammary artery and the internal thoracic artery are the same thing!

22 **D.** Gilbert's syndrome occurs in about 1 in 20. It is more common in males and is an autosomal dominant condition. The enzyme deficiency is glucuronyl transferase. LFTs are usually normal. It causes pre-hepatic jaundice with an increase in unconjugated bilirubin.

23 **D.** *Clostridium difficile* is a Gram-positive anaerobic bacillus.

24	C.	64	A.
25	E.	65	A.
26	D.	66	B.
27	B.	67	C.
28	C.	68	A.
29	C.	69	A.
30	D.	70	B.
31	B.	71	E.
32	B.	72	E.
33	B. This scenario came up in a real	73	B.
	FRCS exit exam. There is great debate	74	C.
	as to the correct answer here.	75	A.
34	B. A Delorme's procedure could be	76	A.
	performed here under spinal anaes-	77	C.
	thesia and may be the safest option	78	B.
	that allows a surgical repair.	79	C.
35	A.	80	C.
36	C.	81	A.
37	D.	82	B.
38	B.	83	B.
39	B.	84	B.
40	B.	85	B.
41	C.	86	C.
42	A.	87	A.
43	D.	88	D.
44	B.	89	B.
45	C.	90	D.
46	C.	91	C.
47	E.	92	A.
48	C.	93	E.
49	C.	94	E.
50	A.	95	C.
51	C.	96	B.
52	D.	97	B.
53	A.	98	A.
54	C.	99	C.
55	C.	100	A.
56	A.	101	A.
57	A.	102	C.
58	C.	103	A.
59	B.	104	D.
60	C.	105	D.
61	D.	106	C.
62	D.	107	D.
63	A.	108	A.

109 D.

110 E.

111 D.

112 D.

113 B.

114 E. The gallbladder normally holds about 50 mL bile. The right hepatic artery crosses in front of the common hepatic duct in about 25% cases.

115 C.

116 C.

117 E. The cremasteric reflex is mediated by the two branches of the genitofemoral nerve. The genital branch is efferent and the femoral branch of afferent.

118 E.

119 E. Normal serum bilirubin is a risk factor.

120 C.

References

- Basse L, Hjort Jakobsen D, Billesbølle P, *et al.* A clinical pathway to accelerate recovery after colonic resection. *Ann Surg.* 2000 Jul; **232**(1): 51–7.
- Best L, Simmonds P, Baughan C, *et al.* Collaboration Colorectal Meta-analysis. Palliative chemotherapy for advanced or metastatic colorectal cancer. *Cochrane Db Syst Rev.* 2000; Issue 1.
- Biem J, Koehncke N, Classen D, *et al.* Out of the cold: management of hypothermia. *CMAJ* 2003; **168**(3): 305–11.
- Binnie NR, Nixon SJ, Palmer KR. Mirizzi syndrome managed by endoscopic stenting and laparoscopic cholecystectomy. *Brit J Surg.* 1992; **79**: 647.
- Bruix J, Sherman M. *AASLD Guidelines on Management of Hepatocellular Cancer Hepatology.* November 2005; **42**(5): 1208–36.
- Csendes A, Diaz JC, Burdiles P, *et al.* Mirizzi syndrome and cholecystobiliary fistula: a unifying classification. *Brit J Surg.* 1989; **76**: 1139–43.
- Dellinger RP. Cardiovascular management of septic shock. *Crit Care Med.* 2003; **31**: 946–55.
- Gurusamy KS, Samraj K. Early versus delayed laparoscopic cholecystectomy for acute cholecystitis. *Cochrane Db Syst Rev.* 2006; Issue 4.
- Hilton R. Acute renal failure. *Brit Med J.* 2006; **333**: 786–90.
- Irving AD, Scrimgeour D. Mechanical bowel preparation for colonic resection and anastomosis. *Brit J Surg.* 1987 Jul; **74**(7): 580–1.
- Koruth NM, Koruth A, Matheson NA. The place of contrast enema in the management of large bowel obstruction. *J Roy Coll Surg Edin.* 1985; **30**: 258–60.
- Leontiadis GI, Sharma VK, Howden CW. Proton pump inhibitor treatment for acute peptic ulcer bleeding. *Cochrane Db Syst Rev.* 2010; Issue 5.
- Marik PE, Zaloga GP. Meta-analysis of parenteral nutrition versus enteral nutrition in patients with acute pancreatitis. *Brit Med J.* 2004 Jun 12; **328**(7453): 1407. Epub 2 June 2004.
- McSherry CK, Ferstenberg H, Vishup M. The Mirizzi syndrome: suggested classification and surgical therapy. *Surg Gastroenterol.* 1982; **1**: 219–25.
- Mirizzi PL. Syndrome del conducto hepatico. *J Int Chir.* 1948; **8**: 731–3.
- Moayyedi P, Soo S, Deeks JJ, *et al.* Eradication of Helicobacter pylori for non-ulcer dyspepsia. *Cochrane Db Syst Rev.* 2011; Issue 2.

- Myrvold HE, Lundell L, Miettinen P, *et al.* The cost of long term therapy for gastro-oesophageal reflux disease: a randomised trial comparing omeprazole and open antireflux surgery. *Gut.* 2001; **49**: 488–94.

- National Institute for Health and Clinical Excellence. Surgical site infection: prevention and treatment of surgical site infection. NICE guideline 54. London: NIHCE; 2008. http://guidance.nice.org.uk/CG74/Guidance/pdf/English

- Parvaiz MA, Hafeez R. Randomized clinical trial of day-care versus overnight-stay laparoscopic cholecystectomy. *Br J Surg.* 2006; **93**: 40–5.

- Peters MJ, Mukhtar A, Yunus R M, *et al.* Meta-analysis of randomized clinical trials comparing open and laparoscopic anti-reflux surgery. *Am J Gastroenterol.* 2009; **104**: 1548–61; quiz 1547, 1562.

- Pizza F, Rossetti G, Limongelli P, *et al.* Influence of age on outcome of total laparoscopic fundoplication for gastroesophageal reflux disease. *World J Gastroenterol.* 2007; **13**: 740–47.

- Rivers E, Nguyen B, Havstad S, *et al.* Early goal-directed therapy collaborative group early goal-directed therapy in the treatment of severe sepsis and septic shock. *N Engl J Med.* 2001; **345**(19): 1368–77.

- Rutgeerts P, Sandborn WJ, Feagan BG, *et al.* Infliximab for induction and maintenance therapy for ulcerative colitis. *New Engl J Med.* 2005; **353**: 2462–76.

- The SCOTIA Study group. Single stage treatment for malignant left-sided colonic obstruction: a prospective randomized clinical trial comparing total colectomy with segmental resection following intraoperative irrigation. *Brit J Surg.* 1995; **82**: 1622–27.

- Scottish Intercollegiate Guideline Network (SIGN). *Dyspepsia.* Edinburgh: SIGN; March 2003, Guideline Number 67.

- Singhal V, Jadhav V. Acute appendicitis: are we over diagnosing it? *Ann R Coll Surg Engl.* 2007; **89**(8): 766–9.

- Solomon SM, Kirby DF. The refeeding syndrome: a review. *J Parenter Enteral Nutr.* 1990; **14**(1): 90–7.

- Stefanidis D, Hope WW, Kohn GP, *et al.* and the SAGES Guidelines Committee. *Guidelines for Surgical Treatment of Gastroesophageal Reflux Disease.* Los Angeles: Society of American Gastrointestinal and Endoscopic Surgeons (SAGES); 2010.

- Turner N, Whitworth C. Edinburgh Renal Transplant Unit Handbook. www.edren.org/pages/handbooks/unit-handbook.php

- Truelove SC. Medical management of ulcerative colitis and indications for colectomy. *World J Surg.* 1998; **12**(2): 142–7.

- Villatoro E, Mulla M, Larvin M. Antibiotic therapy for prophylaxis against infection of pancreatic necrosis in acute pancreatitis. *Cochrane Db Syst Rev.* 2010; Issue 5.

- Wind J, Polle SW, Fung Kon Jin PH, *et al.* Systematic review of enhanced recovery programmes in colonic surgery. *Brit J Surg.* 2006; **93**: 800–9.

- Yeo SA, Chew MH, Eu KW. Systematic review and meta-analysis of the diagnostic and therapeutic role of water-soluble contrast agent in adhesive small bowel obstruction. *Brit J Surg.* 2010; **97**: 470–8.

Index